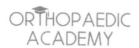

Ortho Quiz

Essential MCQ Practice and Revision Guide

Trauma

Collected by

Orthopaedic Academy

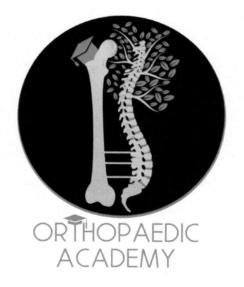

ORTHOPAEDIC
ACADEMY

Ortho Quiz Course

OrthopaedicAcademy

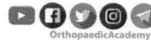

admin@orthopaedicacademy.co.uk
contact@orthopaedicacademy.co.uk

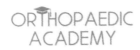

Introduction

Welcome to this comprehensive MCQ Quiz practice & revision guide.
A study tool designed to propel your orthopaedic knowledge and exam preparation.

This guide aims to serve as a robust companion for students, residents, orthopaedic trainees, or any healthcare professional preparing for orthopedic exams.

We have meticulously compiled a wealth of MCQs drawn from a broad spectrum of topics & resources within orthopaedics.

This guide is not just about recalling facts; it's about understanding concepts, clinical reasoning, and applying knowledge.

Each question has been carefully constructed to test your understanding, challenge your thought process, and enhance your decision-making skills. Furthermore, concise but thorough explanations provided for each answer will ensure you grasp the rationale behind the correct choices, thereby solidifying your learning experience.

Whether you're preparing for your exams or seeking to stay current in this exciting specialty, this guide is committed to supporting your journey. We believe the power of continual learning is crucial for any healthcare professional, and our hope is that this guide will be a stepping-stone for your mastery of orthopedics.

Engage with these questions, learn from your mistakes, and above all, enjoy the journey of learning.

Ortho Quiz Course
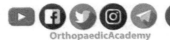
OrthopaedicAcademy
admin@orthopaedicacademy.co.uk
contact@orthopaedicacademy.co.uk

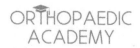

www.orthopaedicacademy.co.uk
www.orthopaedicacademy.net

Index

Design Operations: detailsb2b
www.detailsb2b.com
Email: info@detailsb2b.com

 Raja AL-sahwi
+963967770401

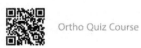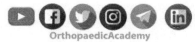

Ortho Quiz Course

OrthopaedicAcademy

admin@orthopaedicacademy.co.uk
contact@orthopaedicacademy.co.uk

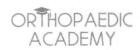

Quiz (1) | Orthopaedic Trauma MCQs/SBAs

1. 25 years old rugby player sustained posterior hip dislocation when several players landed on his back with the hip flexed to 90 degrees, resulting in posterior hip dislocation.
   What is the most common complication of hip dislocation?

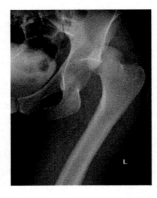

A - Posttraumatic arthritis

B - Avascular necrosis

C - Sciatic nerve injury

D - Recurrent dislocation

E - Femoral artery occlusion

_____

2. A 28 year old man was involved in a motorbike road traffic accident sustaining head injury resulting in a coma and hip fracture.
   Indomethacin is indicated here to prevent which complication?

A - Nonunion

B – Infection

C - Vascular compromise

D - Pressure ulcers

E - Heterotopic ossification

4

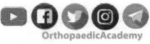

ORTHOPAEDIC ACADEMY

www.orthopaedicacademy.co.uk
www.orthopaedicacademy.net

3. A 33-year-old female basketball player felt a pop and sustained non-contact pivoting injury to her knee when she landed from a rebound. She is complaining of knee pain. Immediate clinical examination shows haemoarthrosis.
What is the most likely damaged structure?

A - Patella dislocation

B - Anterior cruciate ligament tear

C - Posterior cruciate ligament tear

D - Posterolateral complex

E - Lateral collateral ligament

---

4. A 13-year-old boy sustained a tibia fracture following a fall from a swing. The fracture was reduced and placed in above knee back slab in the accident and emergency department. What is the most important early indicating symptom of a developing compartment syndrome of the leg?

A - Decreased sensation in the foot

B - Pain out of proportion to injury

C - Decreased pulses in the foot

D - Inability to move the toes

E - Pale appearance of the foot

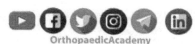

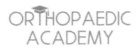

5. A football player fell on his flexed knee with the foot in plantar flexion. On examination, he has a positive quadriceps active test.
    Which knee ligament in most likely injured in this patient?

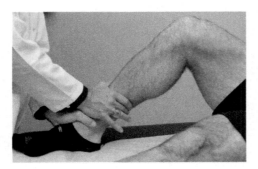

A - Anterior cruciate ligament (ACL)

B - Posterior cruciate ligament (PCL)

C - Lateral collateral ligament (LCL)

D - Medial collateral ligament (MCL)

E - Posterolateral corner complex (PLC)

---

6. A 55 -years-old man sustains an open fracture of the radius which was treated with open reduction and internal fixation. This operation was complicated with radial nerve injury which did not improve at follow up.
    Which of the following treatments will best restore function?

A - Transfer of pronator teres to extensor carpi radialis brevis

B - Transfer of deltoid to triceps

C - Transfer of the flexor carpi radialis to extensor digitorum and the palmaris longus to the extensor pollicis longus

D - Transfer of pectoralis major to biceps

E - Transfer of common flexors tendon to the humerus

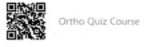
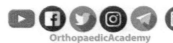

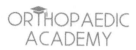

7. A 25 years old man was assaulted with a knife in the axillary region. He presented with weakness of shoulder abduction.
   Which nerve branch of the brachial plexus is most likely to have been transacted?

A - Thoracodorsal nerve of the posterior cord

B - Musculocutaneous nerve of the lateral cord

C - Ulnar nerve of the medial cord

D - Suprascapular nerve of the superior trunk

E - Axillary nerve of the posterior cord

---

8. A 34-year-old male is being resuscitated in Accident & Emergency department following a road traffic accident.
   What is the most important test to assess adequacy of fluid replacement resuscitation?

A - Lactic acid < 2 mmol/L

B - Urine output of 0.25 ml/kg/hr

C - Stability of Glasgow Coma Score

D - Decreased pulse pressure

E - Increased heart rate

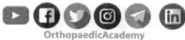

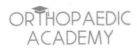

9. Regarding an open tibial shaft fracture in a patient presenting to a hospital without onsite plastic surgery available.
The best course of action is:

A - Resuscitation of the patient and early (within 6 hours) debridement of the wound without stabilisation and plastics review of the patient at an elective clinic

B - Resuscitation and early transfer of the patient to an appropriate specialist centre for combined Plastics and Orthopaedic intervention

C - Resuscitation, debridement and skeletal stabilisation with no plan in place for definitive soft tissue coverage

D - Washout with 2L saline and hydrogen peroxide within resus and plan for formal debridement by Plastic surgeons available within 24 hours

E - Debridement and skeletal stabilisation at local centre with plan in place for transfer to centre with Plastics for definitive soft tissue coverage within 72 hours

---

10. An 18-month-old boy is brought with clawing deformity of his hand. The parents informed that he was born after a difficult delivery by shoulder dystocia. The patient had a right clavicle fracture. A week later the parents noticed the child did not flex the fingers of his right hand. On Examination, his right hand has extension at all the MCPJs of the fingers while his PIP and DIP joints are flexed. His thumb is adducted and is difficult to passively bring it to full abduction. There is obvious wasting of the hand and Forearm. The child can move the arm well with no abnormalities of the shoulder, elbow or wrist. There is no evidence of Horner's syndrome, diaphragmatic palsy, and absent grasp reflex.
The diagnosis of the boy's condition is:

A - Erb's Palsy

B - Cerebrovascular Accident

C - Klumpke's palsy

D - Ulnar and Median combined nerve injury

E – Pseudoparalysis

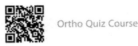
Ortho Quiz Course

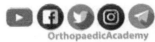

OrthopaedicAcademy

admin@orthopaedicacademy.co.uk
contact@orthopaedicacademy.co.uk

11. In patients with displaced radial neck fractures treated with ORIF with a plate and screws, the plate must be limited to what surface of the radius to avoid impingement on the proximal ulna?

A - 2 cm distal to the articular surface of the radial head

B - 1 cm distal to the articular surface of the radial head

C - Within a 90° arc or safe zone

D - Within a 120° arc or safe zone

E - Within a 180° arc or safe zone

---

12. A 9y old child sustains a proximal tibial physeal fracture with a hyperextension mechanism.
What structure is at the most risk for serious injury?

A - Tibial nerve

B - Popliteal artery

C - Common peroneal nerve

D - Posterior cruciate ligament

E - Popliteus muscle

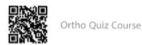
 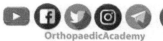

ORTHOPAEDIC ACADEMY
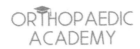

www.orthopaedicacademy.co.uk
www.orthopaedicacademy.net

13. What is the most appropriate indication for replantation in an otherwise healthy 35y old man?

A - Isolated transverse amputation of the thumb through the middle of the nail bed

B - Isolated transverse amputation of the index finger through the proximal phalanx

C - Isolated transverse amputation of the ring finger through the proximal phalanx

D - Isolated transverse amputation of the hand at the level of the wrist

E - Forearm amputation with a 10-hour warm ischemia time

---

14. 36y woman sustained a tarsometatarsal joint fracture-dislocation in a motor vehicle accident. The patient is treated with ORIF.
What is the most common complication?

A - Posttraumatic arthritis

B - Infection

C - Fixation failure

D – Malunion

E – Nonunion

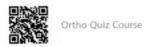
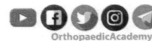

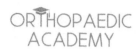

15. What is the most likely complication following treatment of the humeral shaft fracture shown in the figure attached?

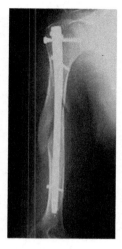

A - Nonunion

B - Shoulder pain

C - Infection

D - Elbow injury

E - Radial nerve injury

---

16. 20y old man sustained a tibial fracture and is treated with a reamed intramedullary nail. What is the most common complication associated with this treatment?

A - Nonunion

B - Malunion

C - Infection

D - Knee pain

E - Compartment syndrome

Ortho Quiz Course

 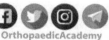
OrthopaedicAcademy

admin@orthopaedicacademy.co.uk
contact@orthopaedicacademy.co.uk

17. A golfer sustained a hook of the hamate fracture. After 12 weeks of splinting and therapy, the hand is still symptomatic.
What is the most appropriate management to allow a return to competitive activity?

A - Continued observation

B - Open reduction and internal fixation of the fracture

C - Excision of the hook of the hamate

D - Carpal tunnel release

E - Guyon canal release

---

18. A 46y old man fell 20 feet and sustained the injury shown in the figure attached. The injury is closed; however, the soft tissues are swollen and ecchymotic with blisters. The most appropriate initial management should consist of:

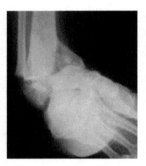

A - Above knee long leg cast

B - Below knee short leg cast

C - Immediate open reduction and internal fixation

D - Temporizing spanning external fixator

E - Primary ankle fusion

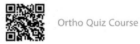   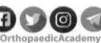

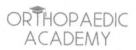
19. A 6y old child sustained a closed nondisplaced proximal tibial metaphyseal fracture 1 year ago. She was treated with a long leg cast with a varus mold, and the fracture healed uneventfully. She now has a 15° valgus deformity.
What is the next step in management?

A - Proximal tibial/fibular osteotomy with acute correction and pin fixation

B - Proximal tibial/fibular osteotomy with gradual correction and external fixation

C - MRI of the proximal tibial physis

D - Medial proximal tibial hemiepiphysiodesis

E - Continued observation

---

20. 13y old boy injured his knee playing basketball and is now unable to bear weight. Examination reveals tenderness and swelling at the proximal anterior tibia, with a normal neurological examination. AP and lateral radiographs are shown.
Management should consist of:

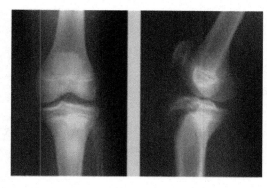

A - MRI

B - Long leg cast

C - Fasciotomy of the anterior compartment

D - Open reduction and internal fixation

E - Patellar advancement

21. Following a traumatic nerve injury, in which time period would a physician find denervation activity with fibrillation and positive sharp waves in the affected muscles:

A - Immediately following the injury

B - 7 to 10 days following injury

C - 2 to 5 weeks following injury

D - 6 to 8 weeks following injury

E - 12 weeks following injury

_____

22. A 25-year-old football player sustained a closed tibia fracture when his planted leg was struck by another player.
Which of the following would be the most common fracture pattern and mechanism:

A - Short spiral fracture — torsion

B - Oblique fracture — uneven bending

C - Transverse fracture — pure bending

D - Oblique fracture with a butterfly fragment — bending and compression

E - Segmental fracture — four-point bending

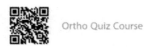
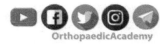

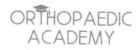
23. Distal one-third clavicle fractures constitute what percentage of all clavicle fractures:

A - 15%

B - 30%

C - 45%

D - 60%

E - 90%

---

24. The most common cause of an indirect injury to the Lisfranc joint occurs through which mechanism:

A - Compression

B - Hyperdorsiflexion

C - Axial load of a plantarflexed foot

D - Supination and external rotation

E - Pronation and adduction

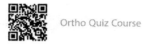 Ortho Quiz Course 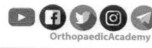 admin@orthopaedicacademy.co.uk
contact@orthopaedicacademy.co.uk
OrthopaedicAcademy

25. After landing awkwardly on his flexed knee, a 22-year-old basketball player has immediate onset of pain and difficulty bearing weight. With the knee flexed 30°, examination reveals increased varus, external rotation, and posterior translation which decreases when the knee is flexed to 90°.
The patient most likely has injured what structures:

A - Posterolateral complex

B - Posterolateral complex and posterior cruciate ligament

C - Posterior cruciate ligament

D - Lateral collateral ligament

E - Posterior cruciate ligament and medial collateral ligament

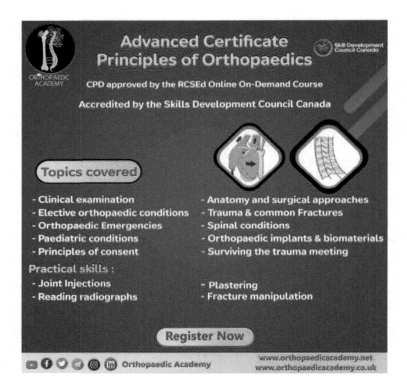
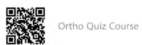
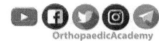

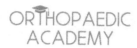

Answers - Quiz (1)

1. 25 years old rugby player sustained posterior hip dislocation when several players landed on his back with the hip flexed to 90 degrees, resulting in posterior hip dislocation. What is the most common complication of hip dislocation?

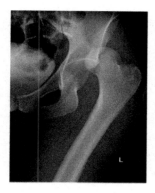

Best answer: **B**
Avascular necrosis

Explanation:
All the above are recognised complication of hip dislocation. Arthritis incidence is up to 20% and is dependent on the severity of dislocation and associated fractures. Sciatic nerve injury is up to 20% and increases with longer time to reduction. AVN incidence is up to 40% and recurrent dislocation is 2%.

_____

2. A 28-year-old man was involved in a motorbike road traffic accident sustaining head injury resulting in a coma and hip fracture. Indomethacin is indicated here to prevent which complication?

Best answer: **E**
Heterotopic ossification

Explanation:
Heterotopic ossification is formation of bone in the soft tissues, may occur spontaneously or following trauma. It is usually not painful but presents with loss of movement. Prolonged ventilation time, brain injury, spinal cord injury, burns, and amputation through the zone of injury in a patient injured in a blast are all literature proven risk factors for development of heterotopic ossification. Prophylaxis is with the use of Bisphosphonates and Indomethacin and raditherpay.Surgical excision could be performed if there is sever loss of movement.

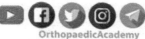

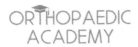

3. A 33 year old female basketball player felt a pop and sustained non-contact pivoting injury to her knee when she landed from a rebound. She is complaining of knee pain. Immediate clinical examination shows haemoarthrosis.
   What is the most likely damaged structure?

Best answer: B
Anterior cruciate ligament tear

Explanation:
ACL injuries are more common in female athletes due to valgus leg alignment and quadriceps dominant control. The anterior cruciate ligament runs upwards and backwards from the anterior part of the tibial spine towards the lateral condyle of the femur. It prevents forward displacement of the tibia. The clinical tests for ACL injuries are Lachman test and pivot shift test. And the investigation of choice is MRI scan. The posterior cruciate ligament runs from the posterior part of the tibia towards the medial condyle of the femur and prevents backward displacement of the tibia especially at 90 degrees of flexion. The lateral and medial collateral ligaments prevent varus and valgus displacement at 30 degrees of flexion respectively.

---

4. A 13-year-old boy sustained a tibia fracture following a fall from a swing. The fracture was reduced and placed in above knee back slab in the accident and emergency department.
   What is the most important early indicating symptom of a developing compartment syndrome of the leg?

Best answer: B
 Pain out of proportion to injury

Explanation:
The single most important symptom of impending compartment syndrome is pain out of proportion to the injury. Children requiring frequent analgesia or complaining of increasing pain should be examined very carefully for possible compartment syndrome. The key word in this question is "early symptom". Pulselessness, paralysis, pallor, and paraesthaesia are all late symptoms and signs. The most reliable sign of a developing compartment syndrome is severe pain with passive stretching of the involved compartment.

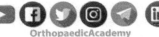

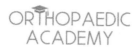
5. A football player fell on his flexed knee with the foot in plantar flexion. On examination, he has a positive quadriceps active test.
   Which knee ligament is most likely injured in this patient?

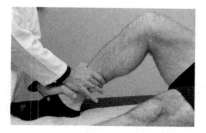

Best answer: **B**
Posterior cruciate ligament (PCL)

Explanation:
The PCL extends from the medial femoral condyle to the tibial sulcus Overall the most common mechanism of PCL injury is a direct blow to the proximal aspect of the tibia such as dashboard injury. The most common mechanism of PCL injury in athletes is a fall onto the flexed knee with the foot in plantar flexion, which places posterior forces on the tibia and leads to rupture of the PCL. Treatment of isolated PCL injury is mainly focused on protected weight bearing, followed with quadriceps rehabilitation.

---

6. A 55 -years-old man sustains an open fracture of the radius which was treated with open reduction and internal fixation. This operation was complicated with radial nerve injury which did not improve at follow up.
   Which of the following treatments will best restore function?

Best answer: **C**
Transfer of the flexor carpi radialis to extensor digitorum and the palmaris longus to the extensor pollicis longus

Explanation:
For radial nerve palsy in the forearm, the most beneficial transfers include transferring the flexor carpi radialis to the finger extensors (to restore finger extension) and palmaris longus to the extensor pollicis longus (to restore extension of the thumb). In radial nerve palsy in the forearm, the patient has adequate wrist extension due to intact ECRL (providing radial wrist extension) supplied by the radial nerve proximal to the elbow. Transfer of pronator teres to extensor carpi radialis brevis, and Transfer of deltoid to triceps are indicated in radial nerve palsy. Transfer of pectoralis major to biceps and transfer of common flexors tendon to the humerus are both indicated in musculocutaneous nerve palsy.

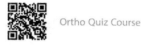 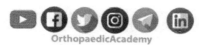

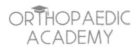
7. A 25-year-old man was assaulted with a knife in the axillary region. He presented with weakness of shoulder abduction.
    Which nerve branch of the brachial plexus is most likely to have been transacted?

Best answer: E
Axillary nerve of the posterior cord

Explanation:
The brachial plexus is formed from the ventral rami of C5-T1 nerve roots. The thoracodorsal nerve of the posterior cord innervates latissimus dorsi. Musculocutaneous nerve from lateral cord supply biceps, coracobrachialis, and brachialis. The ulnar nerve from the medial cord supplies muscles to the wrist and hand only. The supra scapular nerve is a branch of the superior trunk and supplies the supraspinatus. Therefore, will cause weakness of abduction. However, this nerve emerges in the neck between anterior and middle scalene muscles and is more likely to be transacted in neck injuries. The axillary nerve of the posterior cord supplies the deltoid muscle which is the main shoulder abductor.

---

8. A 34-year-old male is being resuscitated in Accident & Emergency department following a road traffic accident.
    What is the most important test to assess adequacy of fluid replacement resuscitation?

Best answer: A
Lactic acid < 2 mmol/L

Explanation:
Rapid fluid resuscitation with crystalloid isotonic solution is the mainstay therapy for hypovolemic shock. Blood replacement is also indicated if the estimated blood loss is greater than 30% of the total volume (class III). Adequate response to fluid resuscitation includes increased urinary output (> 0.5ml/kg/hr), improved Glasgow Coma Score, decreased capillary refill, increased blood pressure, increased Mean arterial pressure, and decreased heart rate. The important blood test is lactic acid, which is increased if the shock is severe enough to cause anaerobic metabolism. Successful resuscitation in a shock patient will lead to a falling lactate level (<2.0mmol/L).

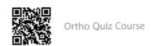 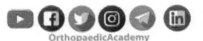

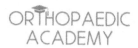

9. Regarding an open tibial shaft fracture in a patient presenting to a hospital without onsite plastic surgery available.
   The best course of action is:

Best answer: **B**
Resuscitation and early transfer of the patient to an appropriate specialist centre for combined Plastics and Orthopaedic intervention

Explanation:
BOAST 4 - guidelines: Although the last option commonly occurs, this is not considered optimal treatment and is only suitable if patient cannot be transferred to specialist centre before need for initial debridement.

---

10. An 18-month-old boy is brought with clawing deformity of his right hand. The parents informed that he was born full term after a difficult delivery by shoulder dystocia. The patient had a right clavicle fracture. On Examination, his right hand has extension at all the MCPJ of the fingers while his PIP and DIP joints are flexed. His thumb is adducted and is difficult to passively bring it to full abduction. There is obvious wasting of the hand and Forearm. The child can move the arm well with no abnormalities of the shoulder, elbow, or wrist. There is no evidence of Horner's syndrome, diaphragmatic palsy, and absent grasp reflex.
    The diagnosis of the boy's condition is:

Best answer: **C**
Klumpke's palsy

Explanation:
This is a case of obstetric Brachial palsy involving C8, T1 (Klumpke's Palsy). Erb's palsy involves upper roots only. Combined nerve injuries can present in a similar fashion; however, low ulnar and Median nerve lesions will not have weakness of FDP and FDS.

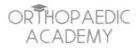

11. In patients with displaced radial neck fractures treated with ORIF with a plate and screws, the plate must be limited to what surface of the radius to avoid impingement on the proximal ulna?

Best answer: **C**
Within a 90° arc or safe zone

Explanation:
The radial head is covered by cartilage on 360° of its circumferences. However, with the normal range of forearm rotation of 160° to 180°, there is a consistent area that is non articulating. This area is found by palpation of the radial styloid and Lister tubercle. The hardware should be kept within a 90° arc on the radial head subtended by these two structures.

_____

12. A 9y old child sustains a proximal tibial physeal fracture with a hyperextension mechanism.
    What structure is at the most risk for serious injury?

Best answer: **B**
Popliteal artery

Explanation:
The most serious injury associated with proximal tibial physeal fracture is vascular trauma. The popliteal artery is tethered by its major branches near the posterior surface of the proximal tibial epiphysis. During tibial physeal displacement, the popliteal artery is susceptible to injury. Injuries to the other structures are less common.

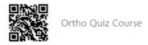
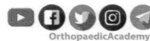

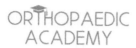
ORTHOPAEDIC
ACADEMY

www.orthopaedicacademy.co.uk
www.orthopaedicacademy.net

13. What is the most appropriate indication for replantation in an otherwise healthy 35y old man?

Best answer: **D**

Isolated transverse amputation of the hand at the level of the wrist

Explanation:

Vascular anastomoses are exceedingly difficult with amputations distal to the nail fold because the digital vessels bifurcate or trifurcate at this level, and little functional benefit is gained compared to other means of soft-tissue coverage. Single-digit amputations, other than the thumb, are a relative contraindication for replantation. Replantations at the level of the proximal phalanx led to poor motion of the proximal interphalangeal joint. In a healthy, active adult, an amputation through the wrist is an appropriate situation to proceed with replantation. Transverse forearm amputation is a good indication with a warm ischemia time of less than 6 hours.

---

14. 36y woman sustained a tarsometatarsal joint fracture-dislocation in a motor vehicle accident. The patient is treated with ORIF.
   What is the most common complication?

Best answer: **A**

Posttraumatic arthritis

Explanation:

The most common complication associated with tarsometatarsal joint injury is post-traumatic arthritis. In one series, symptomatic arthritis developed in 25% of the patients and half of those went on to fusion. In another series, 26% had painful arthritis. Initial treatment should consist of shoe modification, inserts, and anti-inflammatory drugs. Fusion is reserved for failure of nonsurgical management. Hardware failure may occur, but it is clinically unimportant.

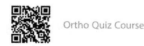
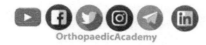

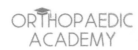

15. What is the most likely complication following this treatment?

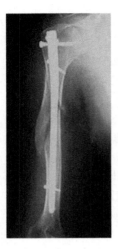

Best answer: **B**
Shoulder pain

Explanation:
Findings from two prospective randomized studies of intramedullary nailing or compression plating of acute humeral fractures have shown approximately a 30% incidence of shoulder pain with antegrade humeral nailing. Nonunion are present in approximately 5% to 10% of humeral fractures treated with an intramedullary nail. Infection has an incidence of approximately 1%. An elbow injury is unlikely unless the nail is excessively long. Rarely, injury to the radial nerve is possible if it is trapped in the intramedullary canal.

---

16. 20y old man sustained tibial fracture and is treated with a reamed intramedullary nail. What is the most common complication associated with this treatment?

Best answer: **D**
Knee pain

Explanation:
The most common complication is anterior knee pain (57%). most patients rate it as mild to moderate and only 10% are unable to return to previous employment. Some authors report less knee pain with a peritendinous approach when compared to a tendon-splitting approach. In one study, nail removal resolved pain in 27%, improved it in 70%, and made it worse in 3%. The incidence of the other complications was infection 0% to 3%, nonunion 0% to 6%, and malunion 2% to 13%. Compartment syndrome is rare after nailing.

Ortho Quiz Course
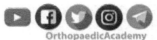

OrthopaedicAcademy
admin@orthopaedicacademy.co.uk
contact@orthopaedicacademy.co.uk

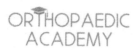

17. A golfer sustained a hook of the hamate fracture. After 12 weeks of splinting and therapy, the hand is still symptomatic.
What is the most appropriate management to allow a return to competitive activity?

Best answer: C
Excision of the hook of the hamate

Explanation:
Excision of the fracture fragment typically leads to rapid return to function. Fixation techniques are difficult to perform because of the size of the bone; hardware prominence is common. Nerve deficits are not typically noted in this injury. The motor branch of the ulnar nerve in Guyon canal must be protected during the surgical approach.

_____

18. A 46y old man fell 20 feet, the soft tissues are swollen and ecchymosis with blisters.
The most appropriate initial management should consist of:

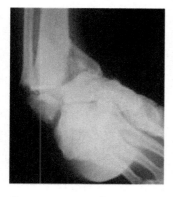

Best answer: D
Temporizing spanning external fixator

Explanation:
Initial management should be consistent of stabilization to allow for soft tissue healing. The use of temporizing spanning external fixation should be the initial step, followed by open reduction and internal fixation when the soft-tissue status will allow. Initial placement in leg cast does not provide the needed stability and does not allow for care and monitoring of soft tissues. In addition, maintaining reduction may be difficult. Immediate open reduction and internal fixation through an injured soft-tissue envelope adds the risk of difficulties with incision healing and a higher risk of deep infection. In the acute setting, primary ankle fusion through this soft-tissue envelope is not indicated.

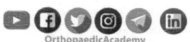

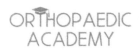

19. A 6y old child sustained proximal tibial metaphyseal fracture 1 year ago. She was treated with a long leg cast, and the fracture healed. She now has a 15° valgus deformity. What is the next step in management?

Best answer: E
Continued observation

Explanation:
The tibia has grown into valgus secondary to the proximal fracture. This occurs in about half of these injuries, and maximal deformity occurs at 18 months postinjury. The deformity gradually improves over several years, with minimal residual deformity. The valgus deformity is not a result of physeal injury or growth arrest. Medial proximal tibial hemiepiphysiodesis is an excellent method of correcting residual deformity but is best reserved until close to the end of growth.

---

20. 13y old boy injured his knee playing basketball and is now unable to bear weight. Management should consist of:

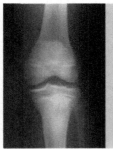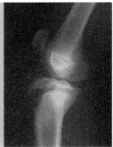

Best answer: D
Open reduction and internal fixation

Explanation:
The patient has a displaced intra-articular tibial tuberosity fracture; therefore, the treatment of choice is open reduction and internal fixation. Periosteum is often interposed between the fracture fragments and prevents satisfactory closed reduction. Most patients with this injury are close to skeletal maturity and therefore, growth arrest and recurvatum are unusual. Non-displaced fractures can be treated with a cast, but displaced fractures are best treated with open reduction and internal fixation. Intra-articular fractures can disrupt the joint surface and are sometimes associated with a meniscal tear; therefore, arthroscopy may be needed at the time of open reduction and internal fixation.

Ortho Quiz Course
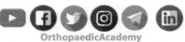
OrthopaedicAcademy
admin@orthopaedicacademy.co.uk
contact@orthopaedicacademy.co.uk

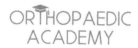
21. Following a traumatic nerve injury, in which time period would a physician find denervation activity with fibrillation and positive sharp waves in the affected muscles:

Best answer: **C**
2 to 5 weeks following injury

Explanation:
Nerve conduction studies can help distinguish between the three principal types of nerve injury: neurapraxia, axonotmesis, and neurotmesis. The following is the sequence of events following traumatic nerve injury: 7 to 10 days - Reduced amplitudes on distal stimulation. 2 to 5 weeks - Denervation changes on electromyographic (EMG) - fibrillation, positive sharp waves. 6 to 8 weeks - Re-innervation on EMG.

---

22. A 25-year-old football player sustained a closed tibia fracture when his planted leg was struck by another player.
Which of the following would be the most common fracture pattern and mechanism:

Best answer: **C**
Transverse fracture — pure bending

Explanation:
A transverse fracture is secondary to a pure bending force. The other patterns included: Oblique fracture — uneven bending: This type of injury typically occurs following motorcycle accidents when the tibia is subjected to uneven bending forces. Segmental fracture — four-point bending: This injury most commonly follows a high-energy injury, such as a pedestrian being struck by a car bumper. Oblique fracture with a butterfly fragment — bending and compression: This is a common fracture that occurs with low- and high-speed injuries. These fractures may occur from car bumpers and motorcycles. Short spiral fracture — torsion: This mechanism is usually from a low velocity skiing injury.

 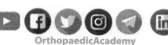

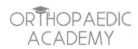

23. Distal one-third clavicle fractures constitute what percentage of all clavicle fractures:

Best answer: **A**
15%

Explanation:
Distal one-third clavicle fractures constitute 15% of all clavicle fractures. The most common location for a clavicle fracture is midshaft.

_____

24. The most common cause of an indirect injury to the Lisfranc joint occurs through which mechanism:

Best answer: **C**
Axial load of a plantarflexed foot

Explanation:
The indirect mechanism of injury involves axial loading of a plantarflexed foot. This type of mechanism is commonly cited in football, basketball, and gymnastics. The most frequent pattern in the indirect mechanism is failure of the weaker dorsal tarsometatarsal ligaments in tension with dorsal dislocation of the metatarsals.

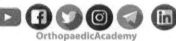

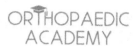

25. After landing awkwardly on his flexed knee, a 22-year-old basketball player has immediate onset of pain and difficulty bearing weight. With the knee flexed 30°, examination reveals increased varus, external rotation, and posterior translation which decreases when the knee is flexed to 90°.
The patient most likely has injured what structures:

Best answer: **A**
Posterolateral complex

Explanation:
With an isolated injury to the posterior cruciate ligament (PCL), posterior translation increases at greater degrees of flexion demonstrating the greatest posterior translation at 90°. Injury to the lateral collateral ligament leads to varus laxity in 30° flexion without posterior translation. With an injury to the PCL and posterolateral complex, varus, external rotation, and posterior translation are detectable at 30° and increase as the knee is flexed to 90°. Isolated tears of the posterolateral complex lead to increased varus, external rotation, and posterior translation at 30° that decreases as the knee is flexed to 90° and the PCL tightens.

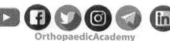

Quiz (2) | Orthopaedic Trauma MCQs/SBAs

1. Following tibial eminence fractures in skeletally immature patients, all the following sequelae have been described except:

A - Residual anterior cruciate ligament laxity

B - Lengthening of the tibial spine

C - Loss of knee flexion

D - Hypertrophy of the tibial spine

E - Loss of terminal knee extension

---

2. A 16-year-old male high school basketball player was making a tackle when he felt sudden pain in his right long finger. He has swelling and tenderness along the volar aspect of the injured digit. He is unable to actively flex the distal interphalangeal joint of the injured digit. Radiographs are negative for fracture.
   Recommended treatment should include:

A - Observation

B - Splinting of the distal interphalangeal joint in extension

C - Splinting of the distal interphalangeal joint in flexion

D - Immediate active range of motion exercises

E - Surgical repair

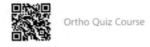
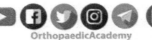

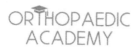
3. A 15-year-old female volleyball player twisted her knee. She states she felt her knee give out. She had immediate swelling and was unable to continue participation. She denies hearing a pop. Physical examination reveals a large effusion with a range of motion from full extension to 80° flexion. She has marked tenderness along the medial retinaculum of her knee. She has no joint line tenderness. There is no pathologic laxity involving the collateral or cruciate ligaments.

The most likely diagnosis is:

A - Partial anterior cruciate ligament tear

B - Partial anterior cruciate ligament tear

C - Medial collateral ligament sprain

D - Patellar subluxation

E - Peripheral medial meniscal tear

---

4. All the following factors have been used to explain why exertional compartment syndrome is more common in the lower leg when compared to the upper arm except:

A - Muscle straining that occurs in the lower leg seldom occurs in the upper arm

B - Muscle compartments of the upper arm blend anatomically with the shoulder girdle making it less likely that bleeding would confine to the compartment of the upper extremity

C - The brachialis fascia is less taut than the crural fascia

D - The brachialis fascia yields more to increased intracompartmental pressure as compared to the crural fascia

E - The pulse pressure of the lower extremity is greater than that of the upper extremity

 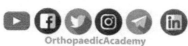

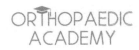

5. A 12-year-old boy presents after being struck by a car. His only complaint is right ankle pain. After obtaining an excellent reduction and casting the leg.
    What are the chances of a significant growth disturbance of his leg:

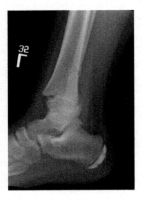

A - < 1%

B - 2% to 3%

C - 10% to 15%

D - 45% to 55%

E - 80% to 90%

_____

6. A 23-year-old man sustains an injury to his foot when falling off a ladder. The foot is grossly twisted inward, and the talonavicular joint is dislocated with the talar head penetrating through the extensor brevis muscle. The dislocation is reduced. The likelihood of this resulting in avascular necrosis of the talus is:

A - Rare

B - 20%

C - 40%

D - 70%

E - 100%

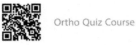
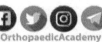

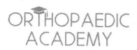

7. A 43-year-old construction worker sustained an injury to his foot 7 months ago. Initially treated with cast immobilization and limited weight bearing. He has lateral foot pain and inability to walk comfortably. Upon examination, pain is present laterally along the course of the peroneal tendons, and no motion of the subtalar joint is present.
The recommendation is:

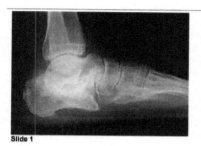
Slide 1

A - Physical therapy followed by job modification

B - Shoe modification and orthotic support

C - Nonsteroidal medication, and ankle foot orthoses

D - Injection of the peroneal tendons with cortisone

E - Subtalar arthrodesis

---

8. A 22-year-old basketball player presents for treatment of a stress fracture of the base of the 5th metatarsal at the junction of the metaphysis and diaphysis. The fracture was treated operatively, and the patient returned to playing basketball. Three months later, it was apparent that a repeat fracture was present. On examination, he has a Cavo varus foot with normal ankle range of motion. Inversion is 15° and eversion is 5°. The base of the fifth metatarsal is prominent.
The most likely cause for the repeat fracture is:

A - Abnormal ankle biomechanics

B - Chronic unrecognized ankle instability

C - Varus heel

D - Bone sclerosis of the fifth metatarsal base

E - Chronic avascularity of the fifth metatarsal base

33

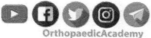

9. Which of the following structures is disrupted in patients with an acute medial subtalar dislocation?

A - Lisfranc ligament

B - Long plantar ligament

C - Talocalcaneal ligament

D - Calcaneonavicular ligament

E - Anterior inferior talofibular ligament

_____

10. Which of the following is not consistent with a complete rupture of the Achilles tendon?

A - A palpable defect 3 cm to 4 cm proximal to the Achilles insertion

B - Ability to plantarflex the foot against gravity

C - Sensation of being kicked in the calf

D - Plantarflexion of the foot with the Thompson test

E - No previous symptoms of Achilles related pain

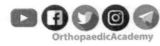

ORTHOPAEDIC
ACADEMY
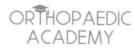

www.orthopaedicacademy.co.uk
www.orthopaedicacademy.net

11. A magnetic resonance image (MRI) of a 15-year-old female volleyball player who twisted her knee is shown . Despite 6 weeks of rehabilitation, she has been unable to return to volleyball without having her knee give out.
What is the most appropriate treatment?

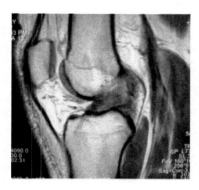

A - Anterior cruciate ligament reconstruction

B - Posterior cruciate ligament reconstruction

C - Continued physical therapy

D - Use of a knee brace

E - Medial patellofemoral ligament reconstruction

_____

12. What is the most common site of pelvic avulsion fracture in a skeletally immature athlete?

A - Anterior inferior iliac spine (AIIS)

B - Ischial tuberosity

C - Anterior superior iliac spine (ASIS)

D - Iliac crest

E - Pubic symphysis

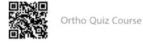
Ortho Quiz Course
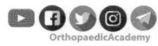
OrthopaedicAcademy

admin@orthopaedicacademy.co.uk
contact@orthopaedicacademy.co.uk

13. This radiograph shows a diaphysis of a 21-year-old female football player. She reported pain in the midshaft of her tibia for 7 months. She has been previously treated with cessation of sports, 8 weeks in a short leg cast, and 3 months of treatment with an ultrasonic bone stimulator.
Recommended treatment at this stage should include:

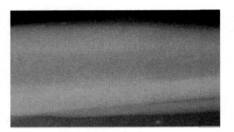

A - Observation

B - Application of a long leg cast

C - Application of a short leg case

D - Continued treatment with an ultrasonic bone stimulator

E - Insertion of a reamed intramedullary nail

---

14. A football player sustains a direct blow to his shoulder. Physical examination reveals ecchymosis over the anterior aspect of the shoulder and painful range of motion. Radiographs include an anteroposterior, scapular Y and an axillary lateral show the humeral head to be located, with an isolated fracture at the base of the coracoid process. Treatment should consist of:

A - Screw fixation of the coracoid base

B - Splinting at 90º of abduction for 6 weeks, followed by progressive range of motion

C - Sling immobilization with gradual progressive range of motion

D - Costoclavicular screw fixation

E - Costoclavicular ligament reconstruction

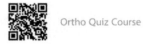
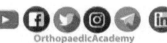

ORTHOPAEDIC ACADEMY
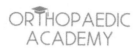

www.orthopaedicacademy.co.uk
www.orthopaedicacademy.net

15. A 56-year-old competitive triathlete fell off his bicycle and sustained a traumatic anterior shoulder dislocation. The dislocation was reduced in the emergency room. No associated fractures were noted.

A magnetic resonance image examination would be judicious in this patient to:

A - Assess the capsuloligamentous integrity of the shoulder

B - Assess for glenoid labrum tears

C - Assess the integrity of the articular cartilage

D - Assess the integrity of the rotator cuff

E - Evaluate the bone for occult fractures

---

16. The initial recommended treatment for a grade 3 acute lateral ankle sprain is:

A - Acute lateral ankle reconstruction

B - Acute lateral ankle repair (modified Brostrom)

C - Functional bracing and rehabilitation

D - Nonweight bearing cast for 3 months

E - Weight bearing cast for 6 weeks

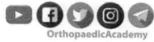

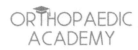

17. Which of the following factors is related to recurrence after primary anterior shoulder dislocation?

A - Type of sport practiced

B - Treatment with immobilization

C - Treatment with physical therapy

D - Patient gender

E - Patient age

_____

18. In the literature, the patella re-dislocation rate for conservatively treated patients ranges from:

A - 5% to 10%

B - 10% to 20%

C - 15% to 45%

D - 40% to 70%

E - 75% to 90%

19. The magnetic resonance image (MRI) of a 16-year-old high school football player who sustained a knee injury during a game is presented. He reports mild swelling at the time of injury but does not recall hearing a "pop." He has attempted to return to football but is unable to make side-to-side movements. On clinical examination, no difference in anterior or posterior laxity is appreciated when comparing the injured knee to the uninjured knee. What is the most appropriate initial management?

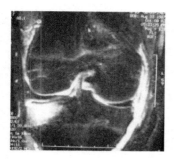

A - Open reduction internal fixation of the tibial plateau fracture

B - Percutaneous fixation of the tibial plateau fracture

C - Medial patellofemoral ligament reconstruction

D - Medial collateral ligament repair

E - Functional rehabilitation with progressive return to play

---

20. What is the most common mechanism of anterior dislocation of the sternoclavicular joint?

A - Medially directed force applied to the lateral aspect of the externally rotated shoulder

B - Medially directed force applied to the lateral aspect of the internally rotated shoulder

C - Medially directed force applied to the lateral aspect of the neutrally rotated shoulder

D - Inferiorly directed force applied to the medial aspect of the clavicle

E - Superiorly directed force applied to the medial aspect of the clavicle

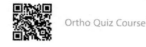
Ortho Quiz Course

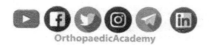
OrthopaedicAcademy

admin@orthopaedicacademy.co.uk
contact@orthopaedicacademy.co.uk

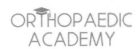
21. A 19-year-old collegiate level volleyball player injured her right thumb during a game. A magnetic resonance image (MRI) through the metacarpophalangeal joint is shown . What is appropriate initial management?

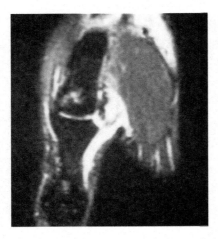

A - Thumb spica cast for 6 weeks

B - Therapy to regain mobility and function

C - Ulnar collateral ligament reconstruction with palmaris longus graft

D - Ulnar collateral ligament repair

E - Excisional biopsy

---

22. After high velocity knee dislocations, there is serious injury to the peroneal nerve in approximately what percentage of patients:

A - Serious injury has not been reported

B - 5%

C - 25%

D - 75%

E - More than 90%

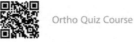 Ortho Quiz Course

  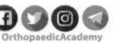
OrthopaedicAcademy

admin@orthopaedicacademy.co.uk
contact@orthopaedicacademy.co.uk

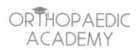

23. When treating recurrent inversion ankle sprains, physiotherapy should be directed at strengthening of which muscle or muscle group:

A - Gastrosoleus

B - Tibialis anterior

C - Tibialis posterior

D - Peroneals

E - Flexor digitorum longus

_____

24. Which of the following is true regarding open fractures:

A - Should not be treated by internal fixation

B - Are associated with accelerated healing potential (compared to closed)

C - Are often treated by delayed primary suture closure of soft tissues

D - Are best treated by saucerization of bone and soft tissue

E - The best time of performing a wound toilet does NOT affect outcome and it NOT clinically important to consider

 Ortho Quiz Course

OrthopaedicAcademy

admin@orthopaedicacademy.co.uk
contact@orthopaedicacademy.co.uk

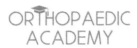

25. A 70-year-old gentleman presents with ongoing pain and poor function to his shoulder following a proximal humerus fracture 2 years previously. Which of the following factors regarding proximal humerus fracture configuration is least likely to be associated with the outcome shown in this patient's radiograph below?

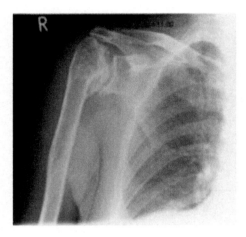

A - A four-part fracture

B - Medial meta-diaphyseal extension of 5 mm

C - 50° of angulation

D - Disruption of the lateral periosteal hinge

E - 1.5 cm displacement of the greater tuberosity

Ortho Quiz Course
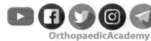

OrthopaedicAcademy
admin@orthopaedicacademy.co.uk
contact@orthopaedicacademy.co.uk

ORTHOPAEDIC ACADEMY

www.orthopaedicacademy.co.uk
www.orthopaedicacademy.net

Answers - Quiz (2)

1. Following tibial eminence fractures in skeletally immature patients, all of the following sequelae have been described except:

Best answer: **B**
Lengthening of the tibial spine

Explanation:
The overall results following adequate reduction of the tibial spine are good to excellent. Loss of terminal knee extension is thought to occur due to hyperemia, subsequent hypertrophy or displacement of the tibial spine and resultant bony blockage. Knee stiffness and loss of extension- very common. Late anterior instability- up to 60%; possibly secondary to ligamentous stretch; unclear whether clinically significant. Malunion can lead to impingement (similar to cyclops lesion after anterior cruciate ligament reconstruction) .

---

2. A 16-year-old male high school basketball player was making a tackle when he felt sudden pain in his right long finger. He has swelling and tenderness along the volar aspect of the injured digit. He is unable to actively flex the distal interphalangeal joint of the injured digit. Radiographs are negative for fracture.
Recommended treatment should include:

Best answer: **E**
Surgical repair

Explanation:
Avulsion of the flexor digitorum profundus, or "jersey finger," is a common injury in sports. Appropriate treatment includes surgical repair.

Ortho Quiz Course

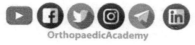
OrthopaedicAcademy

admin@orthopaedicacademy.co.uk
contact@orthopaedicacademy.co.uk

ORTHOPAEDIC ACADEMY

www.orthopaedicacademy.co.uk
www.orthopaedicacademy.net

3. A 15-year-old female volleyball player twisted her knee. She states she felt her knee give out. She had immediate swelling and was unable to continue participation. She denies hearing a pop. Physical examination reveals a large effusion with a range of motion from full extension to 80° flexion. She has marked tenderness along the medial retinaculum of her knee. She has no joint line tenderness. There is no pathologic laxity involving the collateral or cruciate ligaments.
The most likely diagnosis is:

Best answer: **D**
Patellar subluxation

Explanation:
Patellar subluxation is a common injury in athletes. It generally presents with a large effusion. Patients usually have a limited arc of motion but can usually obtain full extension. In addition to medial retinacular tenderness, patients will have apprehension to attempts at lateral displacement of the patella. Treatment is initially nonoperative, emphasizing quadriceps strengthening. Operative treatment is reserved for patients with continued instability despite appropriate rehabilitation.

---

4. All of the following factors have been used to explain why exertional compartment syndrome is more common in the lower leg when compared to the upper arm except:

Best answer: **E**
The pulse pressure of the lower extremity is greater than that of the upper extremity

Explanation:
There are several reasons that have been offered as to why upper arm compartment syndromes are so rare. First, the brachialis fascia is less taut and contains fewer rigid ligaments than the fascia in the lower leg. Second, the brachialis fascia yields more to increased intracompartmental pressure as compared to the fascia of the lower leg. Third, the muscle compartments of the upper arm blend anatomically with the shoulder girdle making it less likely that bleeding would be confined enough to develop into a compartment syndrome. Finally, muscle stresses that occur in the lower leg during events such as prolonged march seldom occur in the arm.

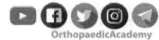

ORTHOPAEDIC ACADEMY

www.orthopaedicacademy.co.uk
www.orthopaedicacademy.net

5. A 12-year-old boy presents to the emergency department after being struck by a car. What are the chances of a significant growth disturbance of his leg:

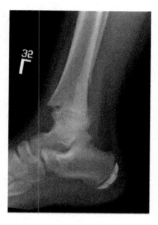

Best answer: **C**
10% to 15%

Explanation:
This is a Salter-Harris type II fracture of the distal tibia. The distal tibia is at moderate risk for growth arrest after physeal injury. The average incidence of growth disturbance is 15% for all physeal injuries in this area. The patient's age and remaining growth also affect the likelihood of a growth arrest causing a significant deformity or leg length discrepancy.

---

6. A 23-year-old man sustains an injury to his foot when falling off a ladder. The foot is grossly twisted inward, and the talonavicular joint is dislocated with the talar head penetrating through the extensor brevis muscle. The dislocation is reduced. The likelihood of this resulting in avascular necrosis of the talus is:

Best answer: **A**
Rare

Explanation:
Medial peri-talar dislocation does not result in avascular necrosis of the talus. The development of subtalar arthritis is more likely.

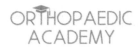
7. A 43-year-old construction worker sustained an injury to his foot 7 months ago. He was initially treated with cast immobilization and limited weight bearing. He has lateral foot pain and inability to walk comfortably. Upon examination, pain is present laterally along the course of the peroneal tendons, and no motion of the subtalar joint is present. The recommendation is:

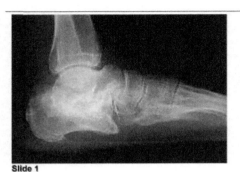

Slide 1

Best answer: E
Subtalar arthrodesis

Explanation:
A worker who sustains a calcaneus fracture must be returned to the work force as soon as possible. Although these alternatives for treatment may be considered in the patient with limited activity and low demands, the longer the time from injury to salvage surgery with arthrodesis, the less likely it is that the injured worker will ever return to gainful employment. Therefore, subtalar arthrodesis should be performed.

---

8. A 22-year-old basketball player presents for treatment of a stress fracture of the base of the 5th metatarsal at the junction of the metaphysis and diaphysis. The fracture was treated operatively. Three months later, a repeat fracture was present .On examination, he has a mild cavo-varus foot configuration with normal ankle range of motion. Inversion is 15° and eversion is 5°. The base of the fifth metatarsal is prominent.
The most likely cause for the repeat fracture is:

Best answer: C
Varus heel

Explanation:
The most common cause of recurrent injury to the fifth metatarsal is unrecognized varus heel deformity. Surgeons must also check for ankle instability, which may be present in this patient. A varus heel, ankle instability, and injury to the fifth metatarsal are associated with recurrent deformity.

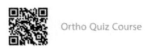 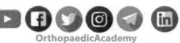

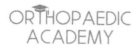

9. Which of the following structures is disrupted in patients with an acute medial subtalar dislocation?

Best answer: **C**
Talocalcaneal ligament

Explanation:
As the foot and the subtalar joint move medially, the subtalar ligaments and the ligaments on the lateral aspect of the ankle are disrupted. The talocalcaneal, or interosseous, ligament is the only ligament that is vulnerable in an acute medial subtalar dislocation.

---

10. Which of the following is not consistent with a complete rupture of the Achilles tendon?

Best answer: **D**
Plantarflexion of the foot with the Thompson test

Explanation:
Patients who sustain an Achilles tendon rupture will often feel as if they were kicked in the back of the leg. They experience the sudden onset of pain and may present with a palpable defect. The patients may note plantarflexion weakness but may demonstrate active plantarflexion of the foot because of other muscles that cross posterior to the ankle such as the flexor hallucis longus and tibialis posterior muscles. The Thompson test (midcalf squeeze) will typically illicit no plantarflexion of the foot.

Ortho Quiz Course
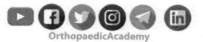
OrthopaedicAcademy
admin@orthopaedicacademy.co.uk
contact@orthopaedicacademy.co.uk

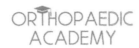

11. A magnetic resonance image (MRI) of a 15-year-old female volleyball player who twisted her knee is shown. Despite 6 weeks of rehabilitation, she has been unable to return to volleyball without having her knee give out.
What is the most appropriate treatment?

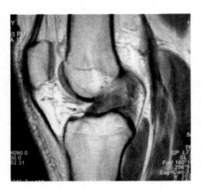

Best answer: **A**
Anterior cruciate ligament reconstruction

Explanation:
The MRI clearly shows disruption of the femoral attachment of the anterior cruciate ligament with characteristic joint effusion. The most appropriate treatment for the patient in this scenario is anterior cruciate ligament reconstruction.

_____

12. What is the most common site of pelvic avulsion fracture in a skeletally immature athlete?

Best answer: **B**
Ischial tuberosity

Explanation:
The most common site of a pelvic avulsion fracture in a skeletally immature athlete is the ischial tuberosity. A pelvic avulsion fracture in a skeletally immature patient is the equivalent of a proximal hamstring injury in an adult. The second most common injuries are to the AIIS and ASIS. Injuries also occur to the pubic symphysis and iliac crest, but they are less common.

Ortho Quiz Course

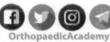
OrthopaedicAcademy
admin@orthopaedicacademy.co.uk
contact@orthopaedicacademy.co.uk

ORTHOPAEDIC ACADEMY

www.orthopaedicacademy.co.uk
www.orthopaedicacademy.net

13. This radiograph shows a diaphysis of a 21-year-old female football player. She reported pain in the midshaft of her tibia for 7 months. She has been previously treated with cessation of sports, 8 weeks in a short leg cast, and 3 months of treatment with an ultrasonic bone stimulator.
Recommended treatment at this stage should include:

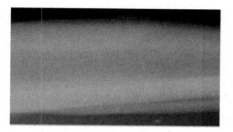

Best answer: **E**
Insertion of a reamed intramedullary nail

Explanation:
The tibia is the bone most prone to stress fractures in athletes. The appearance of the "dreaded black line" is a poor prognostic indicator for healing. Since this patient has failed nonoperative treatment, insertion of a reamed intramedullary nail would offer her the best chance of healing and earlier return to activity.

___

14. A football player sustains a direct blow to his shoulder. Physical examination reveals ecchymosis over the anterior aspect of the shoulder and painful range of motion. Radiographs include an anteroposterior, scapular Y and an axillary lateral show the humeral head to be located, with an isolated fracture at the base of the coracoid process. Treatment should consist of:

Best answer: **C**
Sling immobilization with gradual progressive range of motion

Explanation:
Acute isolated fracture of the coracoid base is almost invariably treated conservatively with the expectation of a good result. If the acromioclavicular joint is sound, the basal fracture is splinted by the costoclavicular ligaments, and displacement is minimal. Treatment with a sling for comfort is sufficient. Pendulum exercises are encouraged. Overhead elevation is restricted for 4-6 weeks to allow healing. Return to a full, painless range of motion usually requires 6 to 8 weeks.

 Ortho Quiz Course
    OrthopaedicAcademy
admin@orthopaedicacademy.co.uk
contact@orthopaedicacademy.co.uk

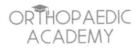

15. A 56-year-old competitive triathlete fell off his bicycle and sustained a traumatic anterior shoulder dislocation. The dislocation was reduced in the emergency room. No associated fractures were noted. A magnetic resonance image examination would be judicious in this patient to:

Best answer: **D**
Assess the integrity of the rotator cuff

Explanation:
Rotator cuff tears may accompany anterior and inferior glenohumeral dislocations. The frequency of this complication increases with age. In patients older than 40 years incidence exceeds 30%; in patients older than 60 years, the incidence exceeds 80%. Shoulder ultrasound, arthrography or MRI is indicated in patients over 40 years of age, with a shoulder dislocation. Prompt repair of these lesions is usually indicated.

---

16. The initial recommended treatment for a grade 3 acute lateral ankle sprain is:

Best answer: **C**
Functional bracing and rehabilitation

Explanation:
A review of 12 prospective studies comparing surgery, casting, and functional bracing with early range of motion revealed 75% to 100% excellent or good results regardless of treatment. The final recommendation was functional bracing.

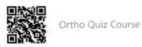 Ortho Quiz Course

OrthopaedicAcademy

admin@orthopaedicacademy.co.uk
contact@orthopaedicacademy.co.uk

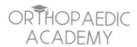

17. Which of the following factors is related to recurrence after primary anterior shoulder dislocation?

Best answer: E
Patient age

Explanation:
The only known factor that statistically correlates with recurrence of anterior shoulder instability is patient age at the time of initial dislocation. The risk of recurrent dislocations is influenced by the age at the time of initial dislocation. In patients <20 years old the rate of recurrent instability is 70–100%, in those aged between 20-30 years it is 70–80% and in patients >50 years old it is 15–20%. The type of sport practiced, type of nonoperative treatment, and patient gender do not influence recurrence rate.

_____

18. In the literature, the patella re-dislocation rate for conservatively treated patients ranges from:

Best answer: C
15% to 45%

Explanation:
**The treatment varies from casting to an elastic bandage and early range of motion.
MPFL is not the only ligament that stabilizes the patella, but it is the most important. Other ligaments that can be injured in patella dislocation include the lateral patellofemoral ligament, the medial retinaculum, and the quadriceps tendon.**

 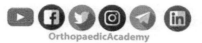

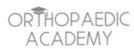

19. The magnetic resonance image (MRI) of a 16-year-old high school football player who sustained a knee injury during a game is presented. He reports mild swelling at the time of injury but does not recall hearing a "pop." He has attempted to return to football but is unable to make side-to-side movements. On clinical examination, no difference in anterior or posterior laxity is appreciated when comparing the injured knee to the uninjured knee. What is the most appropriate initial management?

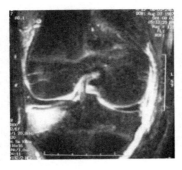

Best answer: E
Functional rehabilitation with progressive return to play

Explanation:

The MRI demonstrates an isolated injury to the medial collateral ligament with an associated lateral tibial plateau bone contusion. Appropriate initial management consists of functional rehabilitation with progressive return to play.

---

20. What is the most common mechanism of anterior dislocation of the sternoclavicular joint?

Best answer: A
Medially directed force applied to the lateral aspect of the externally rotated shoulder girdle

Explanation:

The mechanism of sternoclavicular joint injury may be direct or indirect. Direct injury involves posteriorly directed forces applied to the medial aspect of the clavicle resulting in proximal clavicular fracture and/or posterior sternoclavicular dislocation. More commonly, indirect mechanisms are responsible for sternoclavicular joint injury. Indirect injury occurs when a medial directed force is applied to the lateral aspect of the shoulder. As this force is applied, if the shoulder girdle externally rotates, an anterior sternoclavicular dislocation can occur. If the shoulder internally rotates, then a posterior sternoclavicular joint dislocation may ensue.

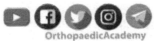

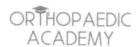

21. A 19-year-old collegiate level volleyball player injured her right thumb during a game. A magnetic resonance image (MRI) through the metacarpophalangeal joint is shown. What is appropriate initial management?

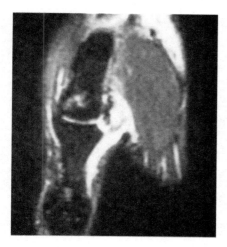

Best answer: **D**
Ulnar collateral ligament repair

Explanation:

The MRI reveals a complete disruption of the ulnar collateral ligament of the metacarpophalangeal joint of the thumb. The preferred treatment for complete disruptions of the ulnar collateral ligament is acute repair.

___

22. After high velocity knee dislocations, there is serious injury to the peroneal nerve in approximately what percentage of patients:

Best answer: **C**
25%

Explanation:

After reviewing several series from 1963 to 1992, investigators found serious injury to the popliteal vessels in approximately 30% of cases and peroneal nerve injuries in 25% of cases. The incidence of arterial and nerve injury with lower velocity mechanisms (some athletic injuries) is lower.

    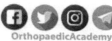

23. When treating recurrent inversion ankle sprains, physiotherapy should be directed at strengthening of which muscle or muscle group:

Best answer: **D**
Peroneals

Explanation:

The peroneals provide dynamic resistance to inversion of the ankle. Therapy programs designed for treating lateral ankle instability must attempt to maximize the function of these dynamic stabilizers.

_____

24. Which of the following is true regarding open fractures:

Best answer: **C**
Are often treated by delayed primary suture closure of soft tissues

Explanation:

this allows the ortho surg to further inspect for signs of infection or muscle ischemia. Other statements are false. Open fracture can be treated by internal fixation provided that the wound has been debrided and irrigated +/- antibiotics prescribed prophylactically. Open fractures show inferior healing potential for obvious reasons relative to closed fractures. Wound toilet should be ideally done within the first 6 hrs since the bacterial colonisation is much less and hence can prevent further contamination by debridement, irrigation + antibiotics. Saucerisation is the Rx of Choice for chronic osteitis, and NOT open fractures.

Ortho Quiz Course

OrthopaedicAcademy

admin@orthopaedicacademy.co.uk
contact@orthopaedicacademy.co.uk

25. A 70-year-old gentleman presents with ongoing pain and poor function to his shoulder following a proximal humerus fracture 2 years previously.
Which of the following factors regarding proximal humerus fracture configuration is least likely to be associated with the outcome shown in this patient's radiograph below?

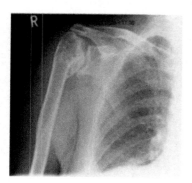

Best answer: D

Disruption of the lateral periosteal hinge

Explanation:

This is a case of humeral head AVN following proximal humerus fracture. The predictors of AVN are four part fracture, angulation over 45 degrees of head, Displacement of tuberosities >10mm, glenohumeral dislocations, head split pattern.

Basic Sciences MCQs

To view the book, scan the QR Code

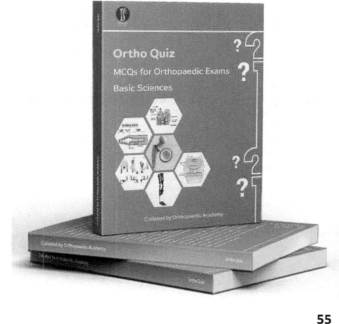

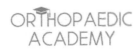

Quiz (3) | Orthopaedic Trauma MCQs/SBAs

1. Of patients treated surgically for patella dislocation, the recurrence rates range from:

A - 0% to 15%

B - 15% to 30%

C - 30% to 50%

D - 50% to 75%

E - 75% to 90%

---

2. 2.A Magnetic Resonance Image (MRI) of the right foot of a 16-year-old female cross-country runner is presented. The patient complains of progressive pain in her right foot. Recommended initial management should include:

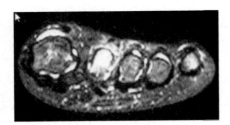

A - Excisional biopsy

B – Non--weight bearing with further workup including nutritional and endocrine evaluation

C - Resumption of activities as tolerated

D - Open reduction internal fixation

E - Incisional biopsy

 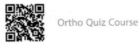   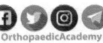

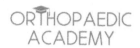

3. Which best describes a type IIA distal clavicle fracture?

A - The fracture is lateral to the coracoclavicular ligaments

B - The fracture involves intra-articular injury of the acromioclavicular joint

C - The fracture line is between the conoid and trapezoid ligaments

D - The fracture is medial to the coracoclavicular ligaments

E - The fracture involves comminuted distal clavicle fracture

---

4. What are the main findings of medial tibial stress syndrome on a bone scan?

A - Delayed uptake of tracer and non-focal uptake over the posteromedial tibial border

B - Lack of uptake of tracer in all phases

C - Focal uptake of tracer in early phase only

D - Focal uptake of tracer in delayed phases

E - Nonspecific uptake of tracer in all phases

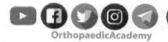

ORTHOPAEDIC ACADEMY

www.orthopaedicacademy.co.uk
www.orthopaedicacademy.net

5. A type 3 traumatic spondylolisthesis of the axis, as classified by Levine and Edwards, is best treated with which of the following:

A - Soft collar immobilization

B - Hard Philadelphia cervical orthosis

C - Halo vest immobilization

D - Open reduction and operative posterior stabilization

E - Gardner-Wells tongs application and awake reduction, then posterior stabilization

_____

6. An 11-year-old boy sustained a fall while jumping on a trampoline. He has moderate back pain, L-5 radiculopathy, and weakness of the right extensor hallucis longus. Radiographs and a computerized tomography scan of the lumbar spine demonstrate a slipped vertebral apophysis. The recommended treatment is:

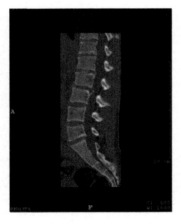

A - Laminectomy and excision of annulus and vertebral bony margin

B - Bed rest

C - Thoracolumbosacral orthosis

D - Physical therapy

E - Spinal traction

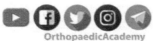

7. Which of the following statements regarding lesions of the spinal cord caused by bullet wounds is true:

A - Twenty-five percent of patients with complete lesions recover one motor level after 1 year

B - Thirty-three percent of patients with incomplete lesions usually have a partial or complete recovery after 1 year

C - Complete lesions occur in more than 50% of all gunshot wounds to the spine

D - 75% of patients in whom the bullet has passed through the spinal canal will experience a complete lesion

E - All the above

---

8. An 18-year-old man presents to the emergency department after sustaining a high-velocity gunshot wound to the umbilical region of the abdomen. An exit wound is found at the L3-L5 region of the lower back. Neurological examination shows grade 0/5 strength in his tibialis anterior muscles, gastrocnemius/soleus muscles, and extensor hallucis longus muscles bilaterally. His quadriceps and hamstrings strength is grade 2/5 bilaterally. A bullet fragment was seen at L4 within the spinal canal on computed tomography (CT) imaging. The patient sustained significant gastrointestinal trauma because of the bullet traversing his body.
Management should consist of:

A - Administration of a broad-spectrum antibiotic for 14 days

B - Removal of the bullet fragment at L4

C - Continued serial neurologic examinations

D - Intravenous administration of dexamethasone for 24 hours

E - A, B, and C

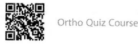
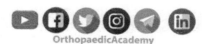

9. What percentage of women with osteoporotic fractures develop kyphosis:

A - 10%

B - 15%

C - 25%

D - 30%

E - 60%

---

10. Comparing manual traction and finger trap traction in reducing distal radius fracture:

A - Manual traction may better correct dorsal tilt

B - Finger traction may better restore ulnar height

C - There is lower incidence of CRPS with finger trap traction

D - There is higher incidence of carpal tunnel syndrome with finger trap traction

E - Manual pain cause less pain during reduction than finger trap reduction

   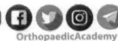

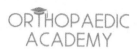
ORTHOPAEDIC ACADEMY

www.orthopaedicacademy.co.uk
www.orthopaedicacademy.net

11. A 55-year-old man with ankylosing spondylitis has a minor fall and is suffering with neck pain. Anteroposterior and lateral radiographs are negative with no evidence of fracture. He has no neurologic loss and has normal strength except for severe restricted motion. Twelve hours following injury, he is found to have bilateral biceps and triceps weakness. The appropriate management and the work up of this individual is:

A - Computerized tomography (CT) anteroposterior lateral radiographs of the cervical spine

B - CT scan of the cervical spine

C - Magnetic resonance imaging (MRI) of the cervical spine

D - Bone scan of the MRI

E - Electromyogram to better delineate all the nerve neuropathy

---

12. Appropriate treatment of a nondisplaced Jefferson fracture is:

A - Hard cervical orthosis

B - Halo vest

C - Soft collar

D - Posterior surgical stabilization

E - Nerve treatment necessary

13. A 38-year-old construction worker fell from a scaffolding and sustains a pure flexion-compression injury to T12.
In this type of injury, which portion of the vertebral body fails first:

A - End plate

B - Subcortical cancellous bone

C - Posterior elements

D - Middle column

E - Lamina

_____

14. Which of the following is the time window from the time of injury during which treatment of nonpenetrating spinal cord injury with methylprednisolone is indicated:

A - 2 hours

B - 4 hours

C - 8 hours

D - 12 hours

E - 24 hours

 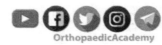

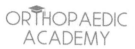

15. Compression fractures of the spine secondary to metastatic disease usually first affect which component of the nervous system first:

A - Balance

B - Bowel and bladder function

C - Light touch sensation

D - Pain perception

E - Motor function

---

16. Which of the following fracture types is the most stable fracture:

A - Teardrop fracture

B - Burst fracture

C - Unilateral facet dislocation

D - Hangman's fracture

E - Clay-shoveler's fracture

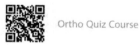
Ortho Quiz Course

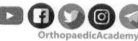

OrthopaedicAcademy

admin@orthopaedicacademy.co.uk
contact@orthopaedicacademy.co.uk

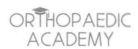

17. A 45-year-old man has neck pain following a motor vehicle accident. His neurologic examination is normal. His plain Radiographs are shown.
The most likely diagnosis is:

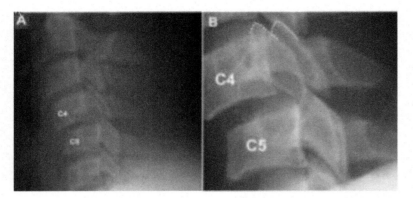

A - Cervical strain (whiplash-type injury)

B - Compression fracture of C5

C - Unilateral facet dislocation

D - Bilateral facet dislocation

E - Spinous process fracture

_____

18. All the statements regarding the atypical femur fracture due to bisphosphonate therapy are true EXCEPT:

A - Fracture is located along femoral diaphysis from distal to the lesser trochanter to proximal to supracondylar ridge

B - Fracture is sustained with minimal or no trauma

C - Complete fracture extends through both cortices

D- The fracture line originates at the lateral cortex and is usually transverse

E - The incomplete fracture can involve either the medial or lateral cortex

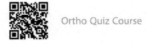
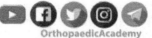

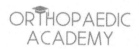

19. Initially, the most appropriate method to evaluate a patient with suspected peripheral nerve injury involves:

A - An imaging study, preferably magnetic resonance imaging (MRI), of the injured region

B - Electromyography and nerve conduction velocity studies

C - A doppler ultrasound to study blood flow to the injured area

D - An MRI of the entire spine to evaluate possible spinal cord injury

E - A detailed neurologic evaluation noting distal motor function

_____

20. Which of the following zones of the physis is involved in Salter Harris Type I and II fractures?

A - Proliferative zone

B - Perichondrial ring

C - Reserve zone

D - Node of Ranvier

E - Zone of provisional calcification

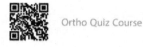
Ortho Quiz Course

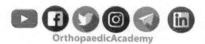
OrthopaedicAcademy

admin@orthopaedicacademy.co.uk
contact@orthopaedicacademy.co.uk

21. A 14-year-old ice hockey player had a jersey pulled over his head in a brawl during a game. He presents the following day with a stiff neck tilted to the right side and an inability to bring his head to a neutral position. On physical examination, his head is tilted to the right 20°, rotated to the left 20°, and slightly flexed. Attempts at passive rotation to a neutral position produce pain. Computerized tomography scans show atlantoaxial rotatory displacement with no anterior displacement of C1 on C2.
Treatment should include:

A - Urgent C1 to C2 fusion

B - Use of a soft collar, exercises, and nonsteroidal anti-inflammatory drugs (NSAIDs)

C - Head halter traction and NSAIDs

D - Philadelphia collar, Minerva casting, and NSAIDs

E - Occiput to C2 fusion

_____

22. The mother of a 4-month-old boy brings him to be evaluated for a swollen leg. The most likely diagnosis is:

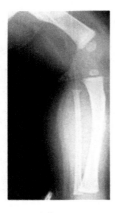

A - Rickets

B - Osteogenesis imperfecta (OI)

C - Scurvy

D - Non-Accidental injury

E - Caffey's disease

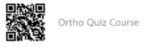
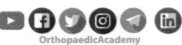

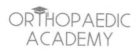

23. Nail bed injury in the adult might be associated with which of the following:

A - Seymour fracture

B - Tuft fracture

C - Fracture of middle phalanx

D - Proximal phalanx fracture

E - Avulsion of central slip

---

24. A 27-year-old banker injured his foot and sustains a displaced divergent Lisfranc fracture-dislocation. The optimal management would consist of:

A - Below knee plaster cast

B - Closed or open reduction and screw stabilization

C - Closed or open reduction and K-wire stabilization

D - A bridging external fixator

E - Closed or open reduction and combined screw and K-wire stabilization

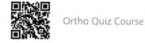
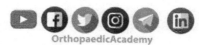

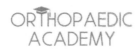 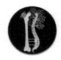
25. A 15-year-old boy sustained an anterior sternoclavicular joint dislocation. What is the preferred management?

A - Open reduction and internal fixation

B - Observation

C - Closed reduction

D - Closed reduction and percutaneous pinning

E - Figure-of-8 brace

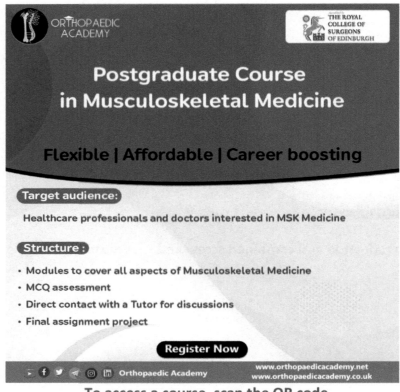

To access a course, scan the QR code

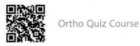
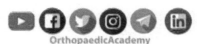

Answers - Quiz (3)

1. Of patients treated surgically for patella dislocation, the recurrence rates range from:

Best answer: **A**
0% to 15%

Explanation:
Of patients treated surgically for patella dislocation, the recurrence rates range from 0% to 14%. The operative procedures have included medial patellofemoral ligament repair or reconstruction, medial reefing, lateral release, and tibial tubercle transfers. The optimal operative procedure remains controversial for first time dislocators. Patients must be evaluated on a case-by-case basis.

---

2. 2.A Magnetic Resonance Image (MRI) of the right foot of a 16-year-old female cross-country runner is presented. The patient complains of progressive pain in her right foot. Recommended initial management should include:

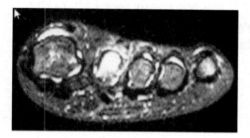

Best answer: **B**
A period of non-weight bearing with further workup including nutritional and endocrine evaluation

Explanation:
The MRI demonstrates a stress fracture of the second metatarsal. Appropriate initial management includes a period of non-weight bearing, as well as assessment of risk factors for additional stress fractures such as poor nutrition and amenorrhea.

3. Which best describes a type IIA distal clavicle fracture?

Best answer: **D**
The fracture is medial to the coracoclavicular ligaments

Explanation:
A type IIA distal clavicle fracture occurs medial to the coracoclavicular ligaments. Type I is an extra-articular fracture lateral to the coracoclavicular ligaments. Type III is an intra-articular injury of the acromioclavicular joint.

---

4. What are the main findings of medial tibial stress syndrome on a bone scan?

Best answer: **A**
Delayed uptake of tracer and non-focal uptake over the posteromedial tibial border

Explanation:
Medial tibial stress syndrome (MTSS), commonly known as "shin splints," is a frequent injury of the lower extremity and one of the most common causes of exertional leg pain in athletes. Medial tibial stress syndrome has a characteristic finding on bone scan of uptake only in the delayed phase. Uptake is non-focal and is along the posteromedial border of the tibia. These findings contrast with a stress fracture, which has focal uptake in the early phase.

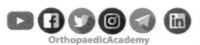

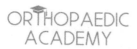

5. A type 3 traumatic spondylolisthesis of the axis, as classified by Levine and Edwards, is best treated with which of the following:

Best answer: **D**
Open reduction and operative posterior stabilization

Explanation:
The Levine classification of traumatic spondylolisthesis or Hangman fractures involving C2. In the type 3 injury has a combined bilateral facet dislocation at C2-C3 as well as the traumatic spondylolisthesis of the axis. Closed reduction could not be performed secondary to the traumatic spondylolisthesis at the C2 isthmus.

_____

6. An 11-year-old boy sustained a fall while jumping on a trampoline. He has back pain, L-5 radiculopathy, and weakness of the extensor hallucis longus. Radiographs and a CT scan of the lumbar spine demonstrate a slipped vertebral apophysis.
The recommended treatment is:

Best answer: **A**
Laminectomy and excision of annulus and vertebral bony margin

Explanation:
This patient has a slipped vertebral apophysis because of trauma. This is analogous to a Salter-Harris type II fracture. A portion of the apophysis and annulus slip posteriorly and may impinge on the exiting nerve root. These usually do not resolve spontaneously or improve with conservative therapy, and excision is indicated. The disk fragments and retropulsed bone must be removed from the canal with a laminectomy for exposure.

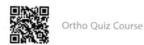
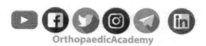

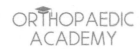

7. Which of the following statements regarding lesions of the spinal cord caused by bullet wounds is true:

Best answer: E
All of the above

Explanation:
All the statements are true. Knowledge of these facts is important in decision-making and management of patients who are victims of gunshot wounds to the spine.

---

8. An 18-year-old man presents to the after sustaining a high-velocity gunshot wound to the umbilical region of the abdomen. An exit wound is found at the L3-L5 region of the lower back. Neurological examination shows grade 0/5 strength in his tibialis anterior muscles, gastrocnemius/soleus muscles, and extensor hallucis longus muscles bilaterally. His quadriceps and hamstrings strength is grade 2/5 bilaterally. A bullet fragment was seen at L4 within the spinal canal on computed tomography (CT) imaging. The patient sustained significant gastrointestinal trauma because of the bullet traversing his body. Management should consist of:

Best answer: E
A, B, and C

Explanation:
Because the bullet entered the patient's umbilical region of the abdomen, significant gastrointestinal damage is suspected. When this occurs, administration of a broad-spectrum antibiotic for 7 to 14 days is indicated to prevent infection and sepsis from gastrointestinal flora. The bullet fragment at L4 should be removed because studies have shown that removal of a bullet from a patient with complete or incomplete neural deficits at T12 to L4 is associated with statistically significant increases in motor recovery as compared to nonoperative management. Intravenous administration of dexamethasone is not indicated for gunshot wounds to the spine because the benefits of steroids do not outweigh the risks.

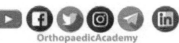

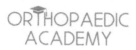

9. What percentage of women with osteoporotic fractures develop kyphosis:

Best answer: **B**
15%

Explanation:

Approximately 15% of women with osteoporotic fractures develop kyphosis. This is often due to the presence of multiple vertebral compression fractures with segmental kyphosis at each level.

---

10. Comparing manual traction and finger trap traction in reducing distal radius fracture:

Best answer: **C**
There is lower incidence of CRPS with finger trap traction

Explanation:

Two primary methods for closed reduction exist and have been evaluated in the literature: manual traction and finger trap traction. Both methods assist the provider to manipulate and reduce the fracture appropriately by restoring the radial length. Sosborg-Wurtz et al6 conducted a recent systematic review of the two methods and noted that reduction by manual traction may better correct volar tilt while finger trap traction may better restore radial length, although these results were not found to be clinically significant. Furthermore, finger trap traction may result in a lower incidence of complex regional pain syndrome (CRPS) and carpal tunnel syndrome and cause less pain during reduction.

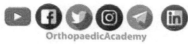

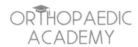

11. A 55-year-old man with ankylosing spondylitis has a minor fall and is suffering with neck pain. Anteroposterior and lateral radiographs are negative with no evidence of fracture. He has no neurologic loss and has normal strength except for severe restricted motion. Twelve hours following injury, he is found to have bilateral biceps and triceps weakness. The appropriate management and the work up of this individual is:

Best answer: **C**
Magnetic resonance imaging (MRI) of the cervical spine

Explanation:
The patient is within 12 hours of having normal cervical spine films.
Approximately one third of patients with ankylosing spondylitis incur occult injuries to the cervical spine that are not identified by plain films prior to kyphotic progression. A bone scan would delineate a fracture after 72 hours. However, the presence of progressive weakness should raise suspicion of a potential epidural hematoma. For this reason, magnetic resonance imaging would better delineate epidural hematoma.

---

12. Appropriate treatment of a nondisplaced Jefferson fracture is:

Best answer: **A**
Hard cervical orthosis

Explanation:
Fractures involving the C1, or atlas are generally caused by axial compression with either a flexion or extension force. Generally, fractures involving the C1 consist of multiple fragments. The classical Jefferson fracture is a 4-part fracture of the atlas and can be unstable. However, in this situation, a nondisplaced fracture represents a relatively stable injury. An open-mouth odontoid anteroposterior radiograph is frequently useful to evaluate unstable patterns. An unstable fracture typically has displacement of the lateral masses greater than 8 mm. If displacement of this amount occurs, generally, the transverse ligament has been disrupted and should be treated by halo vest immobilization. In this nondisplaced situation, a hard Philadelphia collar is the most appropriate form of treatment.

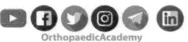

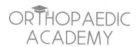

13. A 38-year-old construction worker fell from a scaffolding and sustains a pure flexion-compression injury to T12. In this type of injury, which portion of the vertebral body fails first:

Best answer: **A**
End plate

Explanation:
Failure occurs first at the end plate. The intact intervertebral disk has limited compressibility. Therefore, when the compressive forces exceed the disk compressibility, the load is transmitted to the contiguous bone. The end plate will rupture first followed by the subcortical cancellous vertebral bone.

---

14. Which of the following is the time window from the time of injury during which treatment of nonpenetrating spinal cord injury with methylprednisolone is indicated:

Best answer: **C**
8 hours

Explanation:
Administration of methylprednisolone within 8 hours of injury provides benefit to patients with spinal cord injury. Treatment of patients arriving after 8 hours of treatment has been shown to worsen morbidity. Therefore, patients arriving at trauma centers within this time receive methylprednisolone treatment as part of the standard of care. The exception is the group of patients with penetrating spinal cord injuries where the risk of treatment outweighs the benefits.

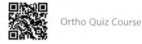
Ortho Quiz Course
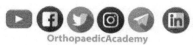
OrthopaedicAcademy
admin@orthopaedicacademy.co.uk
contact@orthopaedicacademy.co.uk

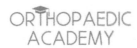

15. Compression fractures of the spine secondary to metastatic disease usually first affect which component of the nervous system first:

Best answer: E
Motor function

Explanation:
When metastatic tumor grows, the posterior longitudinal ligament may be destroyed first and followed by involvement of the spinal cord. Spinal cord compromise can result from direct compression of an enlarging metastatic mass or intradural spreading of the metastatic tumor cells. Retropulsion of osseous fragments or metastatic mass into the spinal canal also may be caused by pathological fracture of vertebral collapse. In compression fractures, the motor function of the anterior part of the spinal cord (anterior corticospinal tract) is usually affected first, followed by sensory loss (dorsal columns) because the spinal cord is located directly posterior to the vertebral body.

---

16. Which of the following fracture types is the most stable fracture:

Best answer: E
Clay-shoveler's fracture

Explanation:
The avulsion of part or all the spinous process that occurs after a violent flexion motion is a one-column injury. The injury is a stable fracture treated by external orthosis, which rarely results in neurologic impairment.

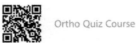
 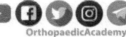

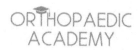

17. A 45-year-old man has neck pain following a motor vehicle accident. His neurologic examination is normal. His plain Radiographs are shown. The most likely diagnosis is:

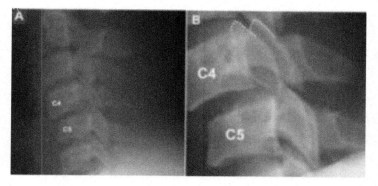

Best answer: **C**

Unilateral facet dislocation

Explanation:

The lateral radiograph shows translation and kyphosis at the level of injury. The facets of C4 do not superimpose on each creating a "double sail" sign. This patient has a unilateral facet dislocation. With unilateral facet dislocations, there is usually 3 mm to 4 mm of forward translation and 5° to 7° of angulation.

---

18. All of the statements regarding the atypical femur fracture due to bisphosphonate therapy are true EXCEPT:

Best answer: **E**

The incomplete fracture can involve either the medial or lateral cortex

Explanation:

The American Society for Bone and Mineral Research task force developed a revised case definition of atypical femoral fractures. Its definition is that of a fracture located along the femoral diaphysis from just distal to the lesser trochanter to just proximal to the supracondylar flare, with at least four of five major features present. These features are: sustained with minimal or no trauma, the fracture line originates at the lateral cortex and is substantially transverse in its orientation (although it may become oblique as it progresses medially across the femur). Complete fractures extend through both cortices and may be associated with a medial spike; incomplete fractures involve only the lateral cortex, non-comminuted or minimally comminuted fractures and localized periosteal or endosteal thickening of the lateral cortex is present at the fracture site.

77

Ortho Quiz Course
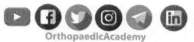
OrthopaedicAcademy
admin@orthopaedicacademy.co.uk
contact@orthopaedicacademy.co.uk

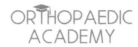

19. Initially, the most appropriate method to evaluate a patient with suspected peripheral nerve injury involves:

Best answer: **E**
A detailed neurologic evaluation noting distal motor function

Explanation:
After a traumatic injury to peripheral nerves, early clinical examination is imperative. The key is to test for motor function in the most distal aspect of the nerve and be able to localize the site of injury. Imaging studies are far more sensitive than clinical examinations. Electromyography and nerve conduction velocity studies are usually performed during the follow-up examination to assess for residual, or recovery of, function.

_____

20. Which of the following zones of the physis is involved in Salter Harris Type I and II fractures?

Best answer: **E**
Zone of provisional calcification

Explanation:
Salter Harris Type I and II fractures occur through the zone of provisional calcification or through the hypertrophic zone. The reserve and proliferative zone remain intact, and growth can proceed normally after healing of the fracture.

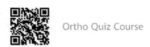
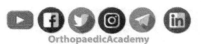

ORTHOPAEDIC
ACADEMY

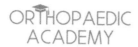
www.orthopaedicacademy.co.uk
www.orthopaedicacademy.net

21. A 14-year-old ice hockey player had a jersey pulled over his head .The boy presents the following day with a stiff neck tilted to the right side and an inability to bring his head to a neutral position. Computerized tomography scans show atlantoaxial rotatory displacement with no anterior displacement of C1 on C2. Treatment should include:

Best answer: E
Occiput to C2 fusion

Explanation:
A soft collar, exercises, and nonsteroidal anti-inflammatories should be tried for 1 week if the diagnosis of atlantoaxial rotatory displacement is made within a week of its onset. If NSAIDs and a collar do not work, a head halter traction administered along with muscle relaxants. If head halter traction successfully reduces the deformity, the patient should be placed in a Philadelphia collar with Minerva casting for 6 weeks. If the patient has no neurologic findings and no anterior displacement, the condition is likely to resolve with conservative measures alone. If surgery becomes necessary, the occiput should not be included in surgical treatment of atlantoaxial rotatory displacement.

---

22. The mother of a 4-month-old boy brings him to be evaluated for a swollen leg. The most likely diagnosis is:

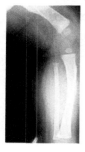

Best answer: D
Non-Accidental injury

Explanation:
This radiograph shows two fractures in different stages of healing. Note the old femur fracture at the top of the field. No evidence of decreased cortical thickness, diaphyseal thinning, or bowing suggests OI. The physis of the distal femur and proximal tibia show no signs of rickets. The presence of fractures rather than periosteal reaction makes Caffey's disease unlikely. The fractures in scurvy are more commonly located in the physis. The diagnosis of nonaccidental injury should be made only after performing a thorough patient history and physical examination.

Ortho Quiz Course
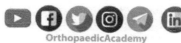
OrthopaedicAcademy
admin@orthopaedicacademy.co.uk
contact@orthopaedicacademy.co.uk

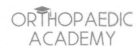

23. Nail bed injury in the adult might be associated with which of the following:

Best answer: **B**
Tuft fracture

Explanation:
Nailbed Injury is associated with tuft fracture in adults and Seymour fracture in children.

---

24. A 27-year-old banker injured his foot and sustains a displaced divergent Lisfranc fracture-dislocation. The optimal management would consist of:

Best answer: **E**
Closed or open reduction and combined screw and K-wire stabilization

Explanation:
The tarsometatarsal joint is best thought of in three columns: a medial column (first tarsometatarsal joint), a middle column (second and third tarsometatarsal joints) and a lateral column (fourth and fifth tarsometatarsal joints). Any dislocation or subluxation needs reduction. A cast or external fixator does not hold the reduction adequately. Although there are many ways to stabilize the fracture-dislocation after reduction, it is generally accepted that the medial and middle columns should be treated with permanent fixation (for example screws) and the lateral column should have temporary fixation (for example K-wires removed after 6–12 weeks). This is due to the relatively greater mobility of the lateral column.

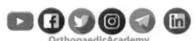
Ortho Quiz Course

OrthopaedicAcademy

admin@orthopaedicacademy.co.uk
contact@orthopaedicacademy.co.uk

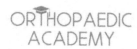

25. A 15-year-old boy sustained an anterior sternoclavicular joint dislocation. What is the preferred management?

Best answer: **B**
Observation

Explanation:

The medial clavicular epiphysis is the last to fuse (age 22 to 25 in men) and sternoclavicular injuries are often Salter-Harris type II fractures in this age group, with opportunity to remodel. Closed reduction is generally not necessary and has a high recurrence rate. Closed reduction is necessary with posterior dislocations associated with compression of the trachea, oesophagus, or great vessels. Figure-of-8 bracing has not been shown to secure a sternoclavicular reduction.

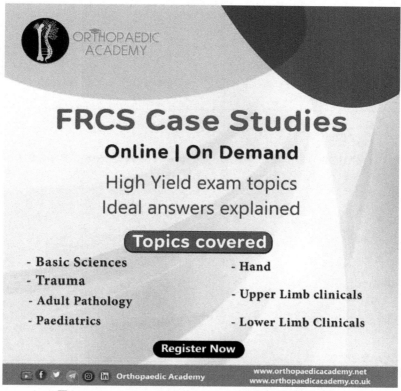
To access a course, scan the QR code

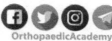

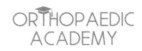

Quiz (4) | Orthopaedic Trauma MCQs/SBAs

1. A 45-year-old man has sustained a minimally displaced spiral fracture at the junction of the middle and distal third of the humerus shaft. He has extensive bruising and swelling of the upper arm, but no open wound is present. He has loss of sensation over the lateral aspect of the forearm and difficulty in flexion of the elbow. Which is the most likely structure involved?

A - Radial nerve

B - Axillary nerve

C - Musculocutaneous nerve

D - Suprascapular nerve

E - Median nerve

_____

2. In humeral shaft fractures, all the following are absolute indications for ORIF except:

A - Open fracture

B - Vascular injury

C - Radial nerve palsy

D - Ipsilateral forearm fracture

E - Compartment Syndrome

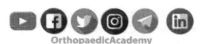

3. Which muscle is affected during the approach to this fracture?

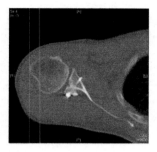

A - Teres Major

B - Infraspinatus

C - Subscapularis

D - Teres Minor

E - Deltoid

---

4. A highly active 20-year-old male, fall on his shoulder while playing Football. Came complaining about pain in his shoulder and limitation of movement in all plans. Which of the following treatments would you recommend?

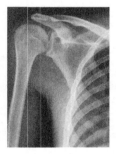

A - NSAID and rest followed by assisted passive exercises

B - Arm sling

C - Open reduction and internal fixation

D - Shoulder abduction cushion

E - Arthroscopic repair of shoulder injury

   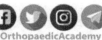

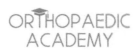

5. 30 years old male suffers from twisting ankle injury. Lateral ankle radiograph reveals a fibular fracture line from postero-inferior to antro-superior.
   This injury can be classified as:

A - Supination external rotation

B - Pronation external rotation

C - Supination internal rotation

D - Supination adduction

E - Pronation abduction

___

6. A 40-year-old male patient undergoes open reduction and internal fixation. 4 months later, he returns with mild ankle discomfort, and a radiograph is shown in Figure. What is the most appropriate next step in treatment?

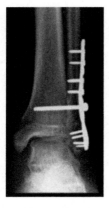

A - Syndesmosis sagittal plane reduction and fixation

B - Syndesmosis coronal plane reduction and fixation

C - Osteotomy and revision of the fibula and syndesmosis

D - Retrieval of osteochondral fragment

E - Revision plating of the fibula and syndesmosis reduction and fixation

Ortho Quiz Course

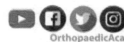

OrthopaedicAcademy

admin@orthopaedicacademy.co.uk
contact@orthopaedicacademy.co.uk

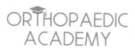

7. For which of the following injuries should lateral pins be placed with the elbow in an extended position?

A - Fracture with the anterior humeral line intersecting the middle third of the capitellum

B – Fracture of the supracondylar region of the humerus displaced anteriorly

C - Supracondylar fractures displaced posteriorly with intact posterior periosteal hinge

D - Fracture with the supracondylar region of the humerus with complete periosteal disruption and instability in flexion and extension

E - Fracture with the supracondylar region of the humerus displaced posteriorly to the humeral shaft with a disrupted posterior periosteal hinge

_____

8. Radiographs of a 32-year-old male shows a lateral malleolus fracture as well as a spur sign on the mortise view. The figure is an axial CT scan of the plafond.
What is the most appropriate treatment of this patient's fracture?

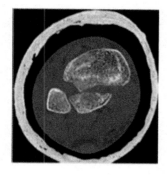

A - ORIF Fibula from anterior to posterior screw placement for posterior malleolus via lateral approach to fibula

B - ORIF fibula, stress ankle and syndesmotic fixation if widening via lateral approach to fibula

C - ORIF fibula with buttress plating of posterior malleolus via posterolateral approach

D - ORIF fibula with buttress plating of posterior malleolus via posteromedial approach

E - ORIF fibula, stress ankle

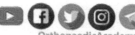

9. A 63-year-old patient presents with right ankle pain after a fall four stairs. The patient reports a history of diabetes mellitus type 2 and peripheral. His injury is reduced and placed in a well-padded bivalved cast. 12 weeks later, the patient presents to the clinic for the first time in the same bivalved cast. The has remained non-weight bearing.
What is the expected outcome at this point?

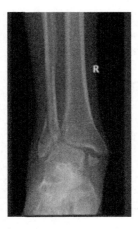

A - Charcot arthropathy

B - Diabetic foot ulcer

C - Deep vein thrombosis

D - Elevation of A1c

E - Fracture displacement

_____

10. What other radiological view, besides an anteroposterior, axillary, and lateral view, would aid in investigation of the shoulder joint in a 25-year-old male who sustained a traumatic anterior dislocation of the shoulder joint for three times in recent 6 months?

A - 30° caudal tilt view

B - Scapular Y view

C - Hobb's view

D - Westpoint view

E - Serendipity view

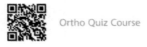
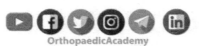

11. A 26-year-old basketball player sustained an ankle injury 6 months prior. He continues to complain of ankle pain and instability.
   What is the next best step in treatment?

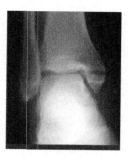

A - Open reduction and internal fixation (ORIF) with autograft

B - Fragment excision

C - Obtain stress radiographs

D - Physical therapy and management of symptoms

E - Percutaneous skeletal fixation

---

12. A 26-year-old male with a BMI of 37 is involved in a motor vehicle collision. He becomes hemodynamically unstable and is found to have the injury shown.
   As well as bladder injury. Which of the following regarding the patient's injury is true?

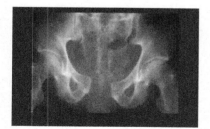

A - His male gender places him at a lower risk for post-operative infection

B - His BMI places him at a higher risk for post-operative infection

C - The mechanism of his injury was likely a lateral compression force

D - The internal pudendal artery is the most likely source of arterial hemorrhage

E - The internal pudendal artery is the most likely source of arterial hemorrhage

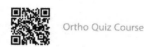
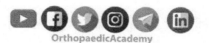

ORTHOPAEDIC
ACADEMY

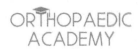
www.orthopaedicacademy.co.uk
www.orthopaedicacademy.net

13. A 42-year-old male presents with severe ankle pain and gross deformity after tripping and falling over. Following fixation of the medial and lateral malleolar fractures, the syndesmosis is assessed and is found to be unstable.
All the following are true regarding posterior malleolar fixation EXCEPT:

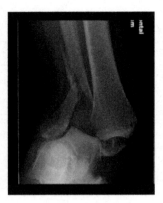

A - Fixation of the posterior malleolus obviates the need for syndesmotic fixation

B - Fixation of posterior malleolus is biomechanically inferior to syndesmotic fixation

C - Functional and radiographic outcomes following posterior malleolar fixation are at least equivalent if not superior to those following syndesmotic fixation

D - Non-anatomic fixation of the posterior malleolus will compromise syndesmotic fixation

E - The syndesmosis is often incompletely injured in the setting of posterior malleolar fracture

---

14. The risk of nonunion in fracture of clavicle which are treated conservatively is increased by all except:

A - Fractures of the lateral end of the clavicle

B - Comminution

C - Complete displacement

D - Male gender

E - Advancing age

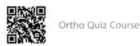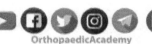

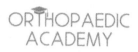
15. A football player presents with severe right ankle pain and inability to bear weight after sustaining a slide-tackle injury during a game. Following medial malleolar fixation, the syndesmosis is addressed.
All the following are true EXCEPT:

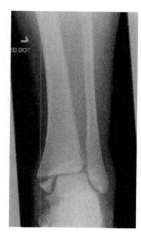

A - The axis of the reduction clamp should parallel the anatomic trans-syndesmotic angle

B - The lateral tine of the clamp should be seated just posterior to the lateral malleolar ridge

C - The medial tine should be placed on the anterior third of the tibia

D - The reduction clamp should be placed 1-2cm proximal to the tibial plafond

E - The surgeon should avoid over-compression of the syndesmosis

_____

16. Which one of the following interventions is not appropriate for a polytrauma patient who has started bleeding significantly from his surgical wounds two days after major surgery and who has been suspected of having disseminated intravascular coagulopathy?

A - Requesting global coagulation tests

B - Administration of platelets

C - Immediate wound exploration and surgical haemostasis

D - Administration of clotting factors

E - Looking for signs of sepsis or systemic inflammatory response syndrome

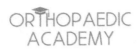
ORTHOPAEDIC
ACADEMY

www.orthopaedicacademy.co.uk
www.orthopaedicacademy.net

17. A 35-year-old morbidly obese female presents with global right ankle pain and significant swelling after a misstep over one of her cats on the stairs. She is unable to bear weight, but the skin is intact.
What is the internervous plane through which direct anatomic reduction and fixation of both fractures could best be achieved?

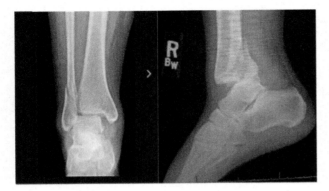

A - Deep peroneal nerve, sural nerve

B - Deep peroneal nerve, tibial nerve

C - Superficial and deep peroneal nerves

D - Superficial peroneal nerve, tibial nerve

E - There is no true internervous plane

---

18. During internal fixation of fractures of the 5th metatarsal, which nerve is most injured?

A - Deep peroneal nerve

B - Dorsolateral branch of the sural nerve

C - Intermediate dorsal cutaneous nerve

D - Medial plantar nerve

E - Lateral plantar nerve

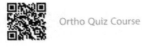

19. A man involved in road traffic accident 5 months ago. sustained open fracture distal both bones of Rt leg. He was treated by washout, closed reduction, and IM nailing. at 3 months, He is complaining of flexion deformity at right big toe.
What's the most probably reason for big toe flexion deformity?

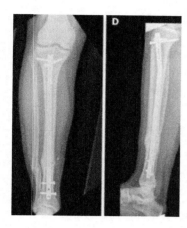

A - Rt Extensor hallucis tendon injury

B - Missed compartment syndrome of anterior compartment

C - Rt long flexor hallucis entrapment at fracture side

D - Limited range motion of rt ankle

E - None of above

_____

20. A 25-year-old man was involved in an RTA. The paramedics reported that his knee was dislocated and reduced on the scene. On examination there was reduced sensation on the dorsum of his foot and dorsalis pedis was palpable. Radiographs did not reveal fractures. What investigation would you request at this stage?

A - Angiogram

B - MRI scan

C - Compartment pressure monitoring

D - EMG

E - CT scan

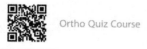
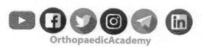

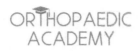

21. All the following concerning hemiarthroplasty of the hip for fracture is true except:

A - Cemented implants are associated with a lower peri-operative fracture rate

B - Cemented implants are associated with a lower overall reoperation rate

C - Cemented implants in general are associated with less pain on mobilisation

D - Cemented implants carry the same overall complication rate as uncemented implants

E - Cemented implants have the same survivorship as uncemented implants

_____

22. Which nerve injury is the supracondylar fractures in children most associated with?

A - Ulnar nerve palsy

B - Median nerve palsy

C - Posterior interosseous nerve palsy

D - Radial nerve palsy

E - Anterior interosseous nerve palsy

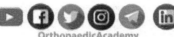

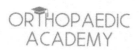

23. Among the following, which one is not a risk factor for quadriceps tendon rupture?

A - Diabetes

B - Gout

C - Rheumatoid arthritis

D - Chronic renal failure

E - Sickle cell disease

---

24. The most significant risk factor for the nonunion of fractures of the middle third of the clavicle among the following is:

A - Smoking

B - Open fractures

C - Comminution at the fracture site

D - Shortening of > 2 cm

E - Obesity

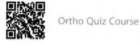
Ortho Quiz Course

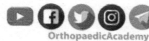
OrthopaedicAcademy

admin@orthopaedicacademy.co.uk
contact@orthopaedicacademy.co.uk

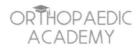

25. Which of the following fractures cannot be treated with Sarmiento functional cast brace?

A - Open fractures

B - Multi-fragmentary fractures

C - Fractures with neurological involvement

D - Fractures with angular instability

E - Fractures with axial instability

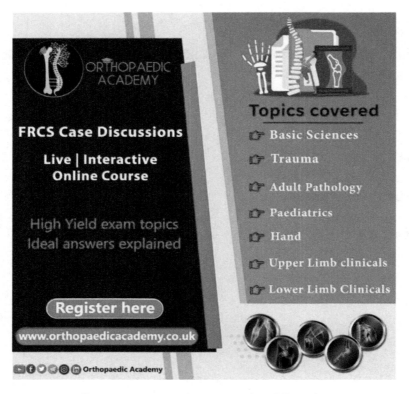

To access a course, scan the QR code

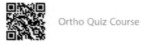
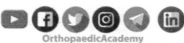

Answers - Quiz (4)

1. A 45-year-old man has sustained a minimally displaced spiral fracture at the junction of the middle and distal third of the humerus shaft. He has extensive bruising and swelling of the upper arm, but no open wound is present. He has loss of sensation over the lateral aspect of the forearm and difficulty in flexion of the elbow.
   Which is the most likely structure involved?

Best answer: C
Musculocutaneous nerve

Explanation:
Musculocutaneous nerve supplies the flexors of the elbow namely; Biceps and Brachialis and other muscle is coracobrachialis. Sensory innervation is a lateral aspect of forearm.

---

2. In humeral shaft fractures, all the following are absolute indications for ORIF except:

Best answer: C
Radial nerve palsy

Explanation:
Radial nerve palsy - as a neurologic injury - is not an indication for ORIF, and patient can be treated with functional brace. While Brachial plexus injury is an absolute indication for ORIF.

Ortho Quiz Course

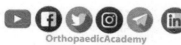

OrthopaedicAcademy

admin@orthopaedicacademy.co.uk
contact@orthopaedicacademy.co.uk

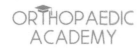

3. Which muscle is affected during the approach to this fracture?

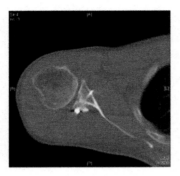

Best answer: **D**
Teres Minor

Explanation:
Teres Minor this a posterior rim fracture of glenoid the most appropriate approach is the posterior approach which goes through internervous plane between the suprascapular nerve and axillary nerve which travels with the posterior circumflex humeral artery which supply Teres Minor. Teres Major is supplied by lower subscapular nerve.

---

4. A highly active 20-year-old male, fall on his shoulder while playing Football.
   Which of the following treatments would you recommend?

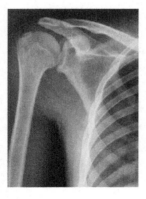

Best answer: **C**
Open reduction and internal fixation

Explanation:
In young active patient with greater tuberosity fracture , open reduction and internal fixation of greater tuberosity avulsion fracture the best treatment plan ,although arthroscopic reduction and fixation can be consider but it is technically challenging in acute phase due to difficult visibility especially with significant bleeding.

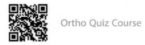
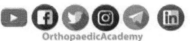

5. **30 years old male suffers from twisting ankle injury. Lateral ankle radiograph reveals a fibular fracture line from posterior inferior to anterosuperior.**
   This injury can be classified as:

Best answer: **B**
Pronation external rotation

Explanation:
Lauge-Hansen ankle fractures classification is based on experimentally created mechanisms.

Lauge-Hansen emphasized the influence that the position of the foot had on the injury pattern and correlated this position with the direction of the deforming forces. The pattern of the fibula fracture can be used to determine the type of fracture. Supination external rotation results in a spiral fracture from anteroinfrior to posterosuperior. supination adduction results in a transverse at or below the level of the joint. Pronation abduction results in a transverse fracture at or above the level of the joint. pronation external rotation results in a spiral fracture from posteroinfrior to anterosuperior.

---

6. **A 40-year-old male patient sustains a bimalleolar ankle fracture and undergoes ORIF. 4 months later, he returns for follow-up with mild ankle discomfort.**
   What is the most appropriate next step in treatment?

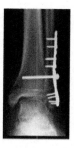

Best answer: **C**
Osteotomy and revision of the fibula and syndesmosis

Explanation:
This patient has undergone ORIF of the lateral malleolus with shortening of the lateral malleolus and lateral tibiotalar tilt. Revision surgery would entail bone grafting and re-plating of the fibula. Malunion of the fibula component of ankle fractures lead to tibiotalar instability and post-traumatic ankle arthritis. The distal fragment is usually shortened and externally rotated. The osteotomy can restore length and correct rotation. Markers for potential instability include: (1) asymmetry of the medial-lateral clear spaces, (2) talar tilt >2mm, (3) talar subluxation, (4) abnormal talocrural angle.

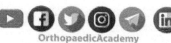

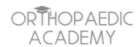

7. For which of the following injuries should lateral pins be placed with the elbow in an extended position?

Best answer: **B**
Fracture with the supracondylar region of the humerus displaced anteriorly to the humeral shaft

Explanation:
Flexion-type supracondylar humerus fractures are rare injuries. They are usually treated operatively and are more likely to require an open reduction given their displacement pattern. They are also more likely to cause injury to the ulnar nerve with the posterior displacement of the shaft. For flexion-type injuries, pinning should be performed with the elbow in extension. For extension-type injuries, pinning should be performed with the elbow in a flexed position.

_____

8. Radiographs of a 32-year-old male shows a lateral malleolus fracture as well as a spur sign on the mortise view. The figure is an axial CT scan of the plafond.
    What is the most appropriate treatment of this patient's fracture?

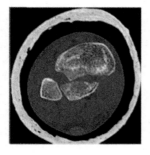

Best answer: **C**
ORIF fibula with buttress plating of posterior malleolus via posterolateral approach

Explanation:
This patient has an ankle fracture with a large posterior malleolus fragment. A posterolateral approach should be utilized for concomitant fixation of the fibula and posterior malleolus. An ankle fracture with a "spur sign" demonstrated on the anteroposterior radiograph is characterized by double cortical density at the inferomedial tibial metaphysis and is pathognomonic for a hyperflexion ankle fracture variant.

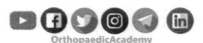

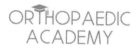

9. A 63-year-old patient presents with ankle pain after a fall. He has diabetes. 12 weeks later, he presents for the first time still in the same cast .
   What is the expected outcome at this point?

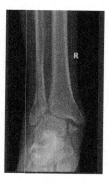

Best answer: E
Fracture displacement

Explanation:
The patient is a diabetic with poorly controlled blood sugar and peripheral neuropathy presenting with a bimalleolar ankle fracture with a loss to follow-up for 3 months. All the answer choices are potential complications with non-operative treatment, but fracture displacement is the most likely to occur.

---

10. What other radiological view, besides an anteroposterior, axillary, and lateral view, would aid in investigation of the shoulder joint in a 25-year-old male who sustained a traumatic anterior dislocation of the shoulder joint for three times in recent 6 months?

Best answer: D
Westpoint view

Explanation:
Westpoint view is good for assessing glenoid bone loss. For a Hill-Sachs lesion, other views could be useful including Stryker view.

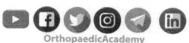

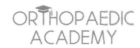

11. A 26-year-old male recreational basketball player sustained an ankle injury 6 months prior. He continues to complain of ankle pain and instability.
What is the next best step in treatment?

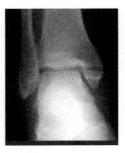

Best answer: **A**

Open reduction and internal fixation (ORIF) with autograft

Explanation:

This patient sustained a medial malleolar fracture that went on to nonunion. The next best step in treatment would be ORIF with autograft.

---

12. A 26-year-old male with a BMI of 37 is involved in an RTA and hemodynamically unstable.
Which of the following statements regarding the patient's injury is true?

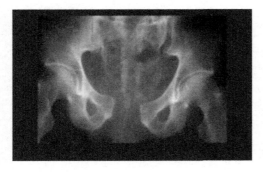

Best answer: **B**

His BMI places him at a higher risk for post-operative infection

Explanation:

Gender has not been found to affect the risk of post-operative infection. The patient's mechanism of injury was likely an anterior-posterior compression force, not a lateral compression force. The superior gluteal artery is the most likely source of arterial hemorrhage in patients with APC pelvic fractures, while the internal pudendal artery or obturator artery is the most likely source of hemorrhage in patients with LC pelvic fractures. Urogenital injury is not a contraindication for pelvic binder placement

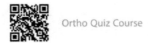
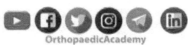

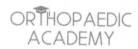

13. A 42-year-old male presents with ankle injury after tripping and falling. Following fixation of the medial & lateral malleolar fractures, the syndesmosis is found to be unstable. All the following are true regarding posterior malleolar fixation EXCEPT:

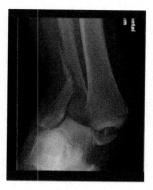

Best answer: A

Fixation of the posterior malleolus obviates the need for syndesmotic fixation in most cases

Explanation:

Fixation of the posterior malleolus has been shown to be biomechanically superior to single-screw trans-articular syndesmotic fixation. Anatomic reduction and fixation will most often obviate the need for syndesmotic fixation, as the posterior inferior tibiofibular ligament (PITFL) is typically intact and attached to the fragment. Fixation of the posterior malleolus has been shown to adequately restore syndesmotic stability and obviate the need for additional trans-articular syndesmotic screw fixation in most cases. Studies comparing clinical and functional outcomes following posterior malleolar and syndesmotic fixation have shown equivalent results with improved maintenance of radiographic syndesmotic reduction following posterior malleolar fixation. Non-anatomic fixation of both small and large posterior malleolar fragments has been shown to compromise syndesmotic integrity and anatomic syndesmotic reduction. Radiographic studies evaluating syndesmotic integrity via MRI have shown the PITFL to be completely intact or only partially injured in most cases.

---

14. The risk of nonunion in fracture of clavicle which are treated conservatively is increased by all except:

Best answer: D

Male gender

Explanation:

Following a diaphyseal clavicle fracture, the risk of nonunion was significantly increased by advancing age, female gender, displacement of the fracture, the presence of comminution and in lateral and medial clavicle fractures.

Ortho Quiz Course
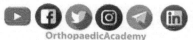
OrthopaedicAcademy
admin@orthopaedicacademy.co.uk
contact@orthopaedicacademy.co.uk

15. A 32-year-old soccer player presents with severe ankle injury during a game.
All the following are true regarding the most appropriate intra-operative technique for anatomic syndesmotic reduction EXCEPT:

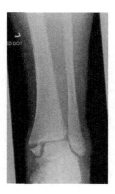

Best answer: **B**
The lateral tine of the clamp should be seated just posterior to the lateral malleolar ridge

Explanation:
The axis of the reduction camp should parallel that of the trans-syndesmotic axis. The medial tine is ideally placed within the anterior third of the tibia, and moreover within the central third of the distance between the anterior tibial and fibular cortices on a true lateral view of the ankle. The clamp is ideally placed 1-2cm proximal to the tibial plafond at the level of the incisura to avoid deformation of the fibula, which has been associated with placement too proximal or distal.

---

16. Which one of the following is not appropriate for a polytrauma patient bleeding significantly from his surgical wounds and who is suspected to have DIC?

Best answer: **C**
Immediate wound exploration and surgical haemostasis

Explanation:
Disseminated intravascular coagulation (DIC) is most commonly observed in patients with severe sepsis and septic shock. DIC is also frequently observed in trauma patients manifesting systemic inflammatory response syndrome (SIRS). DIC is characterized by systemic activation of blood coagulation, which results in generation and deposition of fibrin, leading to microvascular thrombi in various organs and contributing to multiple organ dysfunction syndrome (MODS). Consumption and subsequent exhaustion of coagulation proteins and platelets may induce severe bleeding. In a bleeding patient FFP and platelets may be indicated. The underlying cause should also be addressed.

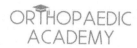

17. A 35-year-old morbidly obese female presents with ankle pain and swelling after a misstep. She is unable to bear weight, but the skin is intact.
What is the internervous plane through which direct anatomic reduction and fixation of both fractures could best be achieved?

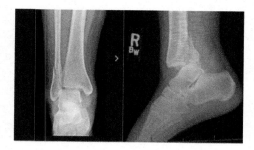

Best answer: **D**
Superficial peroneal nerve, tibial nerve

Explanation:
The posterolateral approach is most appropriate, through which direct anatomic reduction and fixation of both the distal fibular and posterior malleolar fractures can be achieved. The interval is between the peroneal tendons, innervated by the superficial peroneal nerve, and the flexor halluces longus, innervated by the tibial nerve.

---

18. During internal fixation of fractures of the 5th metatarsal, which nerve is most commonly injured ?

Best answer: **B**
Dorsolateral branch of the sural nerve

Explanation:
The standard lateral approach to the base of the fifth metatarsal carries a higher risk for surgical injury to the dorsolateral cutaneous branch of the sural nerve. A "high and inside" approach that remains superior to the superior border of the Peroneus Brevis tendon is anatomically safe and may decrease the chance of intraoperative nerve injury and irritation postoperatively.

Ortho Quiz Course
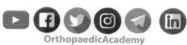
OrthopaedicAcademy
admin@orthopaedicacademy.co.uk
contact@orthopaedicacademy.co.uk

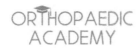

19. A man involved in road traffic accident 5 months ago. sustained open fracture distal both bones of Rt leg. He was treated by washout, closed reduction, and IM nailing. at 3 months, He is complaining of flexion deformity at right big toe.
What's the most probably reason for big toe flexion deformity?

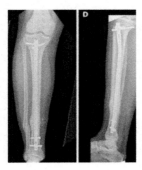

Best answer: **C**
Rt long flexor hallucis entrapment at fracture side

Explanation:
Fracture healing process with callus formation caused catching of long flexor hallucis at fracture side leading to flexion contracture of big toe which is named checkrein injury .

---

20. A 25-year-old man was involved in a road traffic accident and injured his right knee. The paramedics reported that his knee was dislocated and had to be reduced on the scene prior to being brought to hospital. On examination in hospital there was reduced sensation on the dorsum of his foot and a good dorsalis pedis was palpable. Radiographs did not reveal any obvious fractures.
What investigation would you request at this stage?

Best answer: **A**
Angiogram

Explanation:
More than 50% of knee dislocations present reduced. Vascular injury is present in 5% to 15% of patients and selective arteriography in conjunction with physical examination rather than immediate arteriogram is the standard procedure. Peroneal nerve injury is present in approx 25% of patients and up to 50% partially recover.

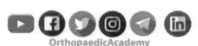

ORTHOPAEDIC ACADEMY

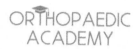
www.orthopaedicacademy.co.uk
www.orthopaedicacademy.net

21. All the following concerning hemiarthroplasty of the hip for fracture is true except:

Best answer: **B**
Cemented implants are associated with a lower overall reoperation rate

Explanation:

A randomised controlled trial comparing cemented and uncemented hip hemiarthroplasty has demonstrated that the general complication rate, including the overall-reoperation rate, is similar between the two groups. The intra-operative complication rate was however higher for the uncemented group. There was no difference in mortality. The cemented hemiarthroplasty group had significantly less pain.

---

22. Which nerve injury is the supracondylar fractures in children most commonly associated with?

Best answer: **E**
Anterior interosseous nerve palsy

Explanation:

The incidence of the nerve injury ranges from 10 to 20%. This presents as paralysis of the long flexors of the thumb and index finger with no sensory changes.

  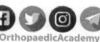

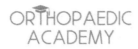

23. Among the following, which one is not a risk factor for quadriceps tendon rupture?

Best answer: E
Sickle cell disease

Explanation:
The risk factors for quadriceps tendon rupture are renal failure, diabetes, rheumatoid arthritis, hyperparathyroidism, connective tissue disorders and steroid use.

---

24. The most significant risk factor for the nonunion of fractures of the middle third of the clavicle among the following is:

Best answer: C
Comminution at the fracture site

Explanation:
Robinson et al performed a prospective, observational cohort study of a consecutive series of 868 patients with a radiologically confirmed fracture of the clavicle, which was treated non-operatively. On survivorship analysis, the overall prevalence of nonunion at 24 weeks for mid-shaft fractures was 4.5%. The risk of nonunion was significantly increased by advancing age, female gender, displacement of the fracture, and comminution ($p < 0.05$ for all). On multivariate analysis, the risk of nonunion was increased by lack of cortical apposition, female gender, comminution and advancing age .

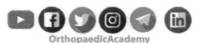

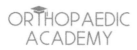
25. Which of the following fractures cannot be treated with Sarmiento functional cast brace?

Best answer: **C**

Fractures with neurological involvement

Explanation:

Functional bracing can be used for fractures that are comminuted, those where axial instability show acceptable maximal shortening and where angular instability is present but can be corrected within a few degrees of normal. Even open fractures can be managed with functional bracing, but this is limited in part by unacceptable shortening and compromise of the soft-tissue envelope required to compress the fracture site.

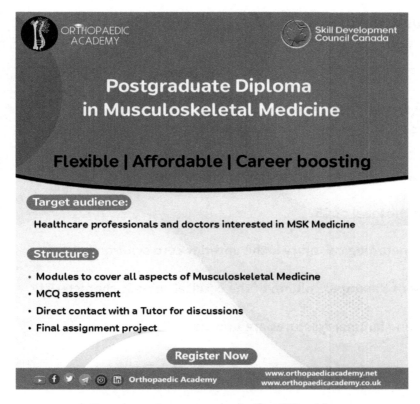

To access a course, scan the QR code

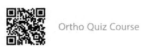 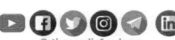

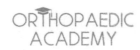

Quiz (5) | Orthopaedic Trauma MCQs/SBAs

1. Which of the following fractures cannot be treated with Sarmiento functional cast brace?

A - Open fractures

B - Multi-fragmentary fractures

C - Fractures with neurological involvement

D - Fractures with angular instability

E - Fractures with axial instability

_____

2. Which of the following statements is not true about the flexion tear drop fracture of the cervical spine?

A - Involves the anteroinferior part of the vertebral body

B - Commonly at the level of C5

C - Characteristic neurological injury is the anterior cord syndrome

D - Displacement of the upper column of the cervical spine is characteristic

E - Sagittal body and laminar fractures are unusual

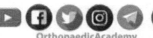

3. Which of the following statements is true regarding the operative treatment of talar fracture dislocation?

A - The deltoid artery provides the major blood supply to the talar body

B - Displaced fractures of the talar head should be treated with open reduction internal fixation (ORIF) using an anterolateral approach

C - 90 % of Hawkins type III talar neck fractures develop osteonecrosis

D - A medial malleolar osteotomy should never be performed as it disrupts the blood supply

E - Osteonecrosis following ORIF of a talar neck fracture dislocation is not detectable radiologically until at least three months following surgery

---

4. A 45-year-old builder presents with a right elbow injury resulting from a fall of standing height. It is an isolated injury with no evidence neurological deficit. You have proceeded with the ORIF shown in the image.
   During the surgical approach, which one of the following statements is CORRECT:

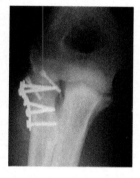

A - The 'safe zone' for posterior interosseous nerve injury exists when the arm is supinated

B - A 'safe zone' for posterior interosseous nerve injury exists when the arm is pronated

C - The internervous plane is between the median nerve and posterior interosseous nerve

D - Involves an intermuscular plane of ECRB and ECU

E - This approach can be extended distally safely

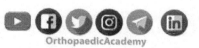

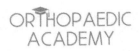

5. What is the greatest determinant of healing after surgical repair of a nerve?

A - Alignment of nerve ends

B - Age of patient

C - Time to surgery

D - Level of injury

E - Sharp transection

_____

6. A displaced fracture of the talar neck with dislocation of the body of the talus but NOT the head would be classified as:

A - Hawkins I

B - Hawkins II

C - Hawkins III

D - Hawkins IV

E - Hawkins V

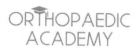

7. A 23-year-old man sustains a dorsal dislocation of the index finger metacarpophalangeal (MCP) joint while skateboarding. Multiple attempts to reduce the dislocation in the emergency department have not been successful. What structure is most likely preventing the joint from being reduced?

Which of the following anatomic structures is most likely to be interposed between the articular surfaces and account for the irreducibility of this joint by closed methods?

A - Volar plate

B - Flexor tendon

C - Extensor tendon

D - Lumbrical tendon

E - Radial collateral ligament

_____

8. A 42-year-old intoxicated man presents after being involved in a fight. On the physical exam, there is a puncture wound with minimal drainage. Had a culture been performed, what would have been the most common organism isolated?

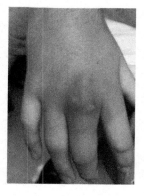

A - Corynebacterium diphtheria

B - Eikenella corrodens

C - Moraxella catarrhalis

D - Pasteurella multocida

E - Polymicrobial

   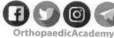

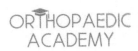
9. The talocrural angle of an ankle mortise x-ray is formed between a line perpendicular to the tibial plafond and a line drawn:

A - perpendicular to the medial clear space

B - parallel to the talar body

C - between the tips of the malleoli

D - perpendicular to the shaft of the fibular

E - parallel to the subtalar joint

---

10. Which one of the following would be the most suitable approach to stabilise a T-type fracture of the acetabulum?

A - Kocher Langenbeck

B - Ilioinguinal

C - Modified Smith Peterson

D - Ilio-femoral approach

E - Combined anterior and posterior approach

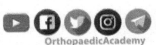 Ortho Quiz Course

OrthopaedicAcademy

admin@orthopaedicacademy.co.uk
contact@orthopaedicacademy.co.uk

11. In a pilon fracture, the Chaput fragment typically maintains soft tissue attachment via which of the following structures?

A - Interosseous ligament

B - Anterior inferior tibiofibular ligament

C - Posterior inferior tibiofibular ligament

D - Deltoid ligament

E - Tibiotalar ligament

_____

12. To be most effective, poller screws should be placed at which location when treating a proximal third tibial shaft fracture that tends to adopt a valgus position?

A - Medial to the nail in the metaphyseal segment

B - Medial side of the nail in the diaphyseal segment

Medial to lateral in the metaphyseal segment posterior to the nail

D - Lateral to the nail in the metaphyseal segment

E - Lateral side of the nail in the diaphyseal segment

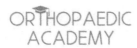
ORTHOPAEDIC
ACADEMY

www.orthopaedicacademy.co.uk
www.orthopaedicacademy.net

13. During cast application, all of the following are directly related to the risk of thermal injury EXCEPT.

A - Dipping water temperature is > 24C (75F)

B - More than 8 layers of plaster are used

C - Fiberglass is overwrapped over plaster

D - During cast setting, placing limb on a pillow

E - Type of fracture pattern

_____

14. Percutaneous iliosacral screw placement will have which of the following likely neurologic complication?

A - Weakness in knee extension

B - Weakness in Ankle plantar flexion

C - Weakness in Great toe extension

D - Decreased Achilles reflex

E - Decreased Patellar reflex

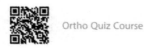
Ortho Quiz Course

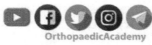
OrthopaedicAcademy

admin@orthopaedicacademy.co.uk
contact@orthopaedicacademy.co.uk

15. The proximal aspect of the posterior approach (Thompson) to the radius involves what surgical interval?

A - Extensor carpi radialis brevis and extensor carpi radialis longus

B - Extensor carpi radialis brevis and extensor digitorum communis

C - Supinator and brachioradialis

D - Extensor carpi radialis longus and brachioradialis

E - Extensor digitorum communis and brachioradialis

---

16. Which of the following statements is incorrect regarding ankle fractures?

A - On a mortise view, the tibiofibular overlap should normally be more than 4mm

B - Maisonneuve fracture is high fibular fracture and involves disruption of syndesmosis

C - Dupuytren's fracture is a fracture-dislocation with a high fibular fracture

D - AP radiograph, the medial clear space should be less than 4mm

E - The talocrural angel can be used to assess shortening

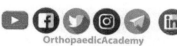

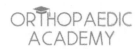

17. When approaching a proximal diaphyseal radius fracture via the Henry approach (volar), the forearm is supinated to minimize injury to what structure?

A - Ulnar nerve

B - Median nerve

Posterior interosseus nerve

D - Lateral antebrachial cutaneous nerve

E - Radial nerve

_____

18. A child is admitted with a femur shaft fracture. You are considering using Gallows traction to manage this injury. Which of the following is a contraindication for your choice?

A - Fracture is transverse

B - The child is 2 years old

C - The child weights 20 kg

D - There is an ipsilateral humerus fracture

E - There is a safeguarding concern

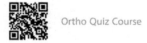
Ortho Quiz Course

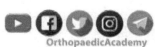
OrthopaedicAcademy

admin@orthopaedicacademy.co.uk
contact@orthopaedicacademy.co.uk

19. A healthy man who weighs 70 kg sustains blood loss of 2 liters after a motorcycle crash. Which of the following statements about physiologic parameters is unique to this amount of blood loss?

A - Pulse pressure will be widened

B - Urine output will be at the lower limits of normal

C -Tachycardia will be present, but with no change in systolic blood pressure

D - Systolic blood pressure will be decreased with a narrowed pulse pressure

E - Systolic blood pressure will be maintained with an elevated diastolic blood pressure

---

20. Which of the following fluoroscopic views is used to assess intra-articular screw penetration during volar fixation of a distal radius fracture?

A - Dorsal skyline view

B - AP wrist view

C - PA wrist view

D - 23° elevated lateral view

E - 45° oblique lateral view

Ortho Quiz Course

OrthopaedicAcademy

admin@orthopaedicacademy.co.uk
contact@orthopaedicacademy.co.uk

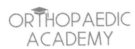
21. A fracture of the radial head is surgically exposed using a posterolateral approach to the elbow. Once the radial head is exposed, how should the arm be positioned to best protect the posterior interosseous nerve from injury?

A - Full elbow flexion and wrist extension

B - Full forearm supination

C - Full elbow extension and wrist extension

D - Forearm pronation

E - Neutral forearm rotation

---

22. When plating fractures of the femoral diaphysis, the plate should be applied to which surface of the femur.

A - Anterolateral

B - Posterolateral

C - Lateral

D - Anterior

E - Medial

Ortho Quiz Course

 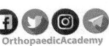

OrthopaedicAcademy

admin@orthopaedicacademy.co.uk
contact@orthopaedicacademy.co.uk

23. Which of the following statements is incorrect regarding ankle fractures?

A - On a mortise view, the tibiofibular overlap should normally be more than 4mm

B - Maisonneuve's fracture is a high fibular fracture and involves disruption of syndesmosis

C - Dupuytren's fracture is a fracture-dislocation with a high fibular fracture

D - On an AP radiograph, the medial clear space should be less than 4mm

E - The talocrural angle can be used to assess shorting

---

24. 65-A patient undergoes open reduction and internal fixation of a displaced radial neck fracture. What position should the forearm be in during the approach and during fixation?

A - Supinated during the approach and neutral for plate application

B - Neutral during the approach and pronated for plate application

C - Pronated during the approach and neutral for plate application

D - Pronated during the approach and pronated for plate application

E - Pronated during the approach and supinated for plate application

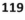

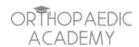

25. What measurement of intra-compartmental pressure could help confirm the diagnosis of an acute compartment syndrome in addition to clinical suspicion?

A - Compartment pressure of 25 mmHg

B - Compartment pressure of 15 mmHg

C - Delta p' of 55 mmHg

D - Delta p' of 45 mmHg

E - Delta p' of 25 mmHg

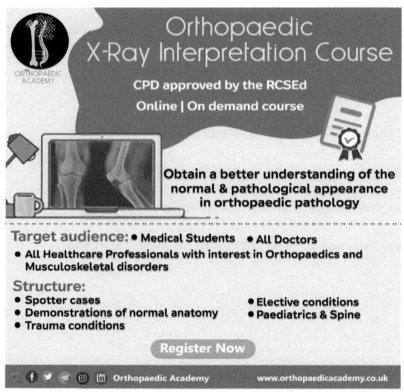

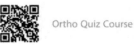

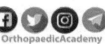

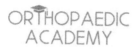

Answers - Quiz (5)

1. Which of the following fractures cannot be treated with Sarmiento functional cast brace?

Best answer: **C**
Fractures with neurological involvement

Explanation:
Functional bracing can be used for fractures that are comminuted, those where axial instability show acceptable maximal shortening and where angular instability is present but can be corrected within a few degrees of normal. Even open fractures can be managed with functional bracing, but this is limited in part by unacceptable shortening and compromise of the soft-tissue envelope required to compress the fracture site.

---

2. Which of the following statements is not true about the flexion tear drop fracture of the cervical spine?

Best answer: **E**
Sagittal body and laminar fractures are unusual

Explanation:
Its name is derived from the characteristic triangle-shaped fragment that fractures from the anteroinferior corner of the vertebral body, resembles a drop of water dripping from the vertebral body. Characteristically there is posterior displacement of the upper column of the divided cervical spine. The injury is frequently associated with sagittal body and laminar fractures. The most common level is C5, and anterior cord syndrome is the characteristic neurological injury pattern.

 Ortho Quiz Course

OrthopaedicAcademy

admin@orthopaedicacademy.co.uk
contact@orthopaedicacademy.co.uk

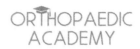

3. Which of the following statements is true regarding the operative treatment of talar fracture dislocation?

Best answer: C
90 % of Hawkins type III talar neck fractures develop osteonecrosis

Explanation:
The major arterial supply is from the posterior tibial artery via the artery of the tarsal canal. Hawkin's sign (subchondral lucency) is best seen on mortise view at 6-8 weeks and is a good prognostic sign. Hawkin's type 3 fractures have an AVN rate of approximately 90%.

---

4. A 45-year-old builder presents with a elbow injury resulting from a fall .You have proceeded with the ORIF shown in the image.
   During the surgical approach, which one of the following statements is CORRECT:

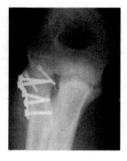

Best answer: **B**
A 'safe zone' for posterior interosseous nerve injury exists when the arm is pronated

Explanation:
The posterolateral approach (Kocher) to the radial head is useful for all surgeries to the radial head and neck. The forearm must be fully pronated to move the posterior interosseous nerve away from the operative field. The posterior interosseous nerve is in no danger as long as the dissection remains proximal to the annular ligament. Pronation of the forearm keeps the nerve as far from the operative field as it possibly can be. The internervous plane lies between the anconeus, which is supplied by the radial nerve, and the extensor carpi ulnaris, which is supplied by the posterior interosseous nerve. There is no way to extend this approach profitably in any direction. Do not incise the capsule too far anteriorly; the radial nerve runs over the front of the anterolateral portion of the elbow capsule. Do not continue the dissection below the annular ligament or retract vigorously, distally, or anteriorly, because the posterior interosseous nerve lies within the substance of the supinator muscle and is vulnerable to injury.

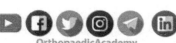

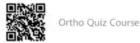

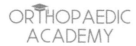
5. What is the greatest determinant of healing after surgical repair of a nerve ?

Best answer: **B**

Age of patient

Explanation:

Age of patient Whereas all answers are important determinants, younger patients have an enhanced potential for recovery.

_____

6. A displaced fracture of the talar neck with dislocation of the body of the talus but NOT the head would be classified as:

Best answer: **C**

Hawkins III

Explanation:

Dislocation of the body of talus but NOT the talus head indicates a subtalar and tibiotalar dislocation with intact talonavicular joint which would be classified as type III Hawkins. Fractures of the neck of the talus based on the modified Hawkins classification are: Type I fracture is a talar neck fracture (AVN 5%). Type II is a talar neck fracture with subtalar dislocation (AVN 18%). Type III is a talar neck fracture with subtalar and tibiotalar dislocations (AVN 44%). Type IV is a talar neck fracture with subtalar, tibiotalar, and talonavicular dislocations (AVN 12%).

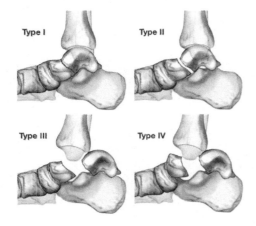

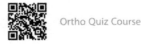
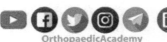

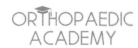

7. A 23-year-old man sustains a dorsal dislocation of the index finger metacarpophalangeal (MCP) joint while skateboarding. Multiple attempts to reduce the dislocation in the emergency department have not been successful. What structure is most likely preventing the joint from being reduced?
Which of the following anatomic structures is most likely to be interposed between the articular surfaces and account for the irreducibility of this joint by closed methods?

Best answer: **A**
Volar plate

Explanation:
The most common structure preventing reduction of a MCP dislocation is the volar plate. It is most easily treated by a dorsal approach and a longitudinal split of the plate. Whereas it has been described that the metacarpal head can become entrapped between the radial lumbrical and the flexor tendon, replacement of the plate volar to the metacarpal head during surgery allows for the joint to be easily reduced with no attention paid to the lumbrical or flexor tendon. The collateral ligaments and the extensor tendon have not been described as structures that prevent reduction of the MCP joint.

---

8. A 42-year-old intoxicated man presents after being involved in a fight. On physical exam, there is a puncture wound with minimal drainage. Had a culture been performed, what would have been the most common organism isolated?

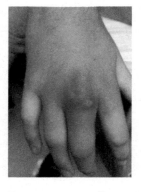

Best answer: **E**
Polymicrobial

Explanation:
This patient has sustained a human fight bite and is presenting with signs of infection. If cultured, the most common isolate is often polymicrobial.

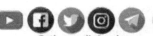

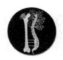
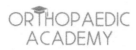

9. The talocrural angle of an ankle mortise x-ray is formed between a line perpendicular to the tibial plafond and a line drawn:

Best answer: **C**
between the tips of the malleoli

Explanation:
The talocrural angle is formed by the intersection of a line perpendicular to the plafond with a line drawn between the malleoli (average = 83+/-4deg).

_____

10. Which one of the following would be the most suitable approach to stabilise a T-type fracture of the acetabulum?

Best answer: **E**
Combined anterior and posterior approach

Explanation:
This pattern combines a transverse component with a stem which exits either through the obturator ring or at various levels through the ischium.

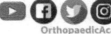

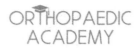

11. In a pilon fracture, the Chaput fragment typically maintains soft tissue attachment via which of the following structures?

Best answer: **B**
Anterior inferior tibiofibular ligament

Explanation:
Chaput fragment (anterolateral fragment of the distal tibia) attaches to the anterior inferior tibiofibular ligament .

_____

12. To be most effective, poller screws should be placed at which location when treating a proximal third tibial shaft fracture that tends to adopt a valgus position?

Best answer: **D**
Lateral to the nail in the metaphyseal segment

Explanation:
As a general principle, the blocking screw is optimally placed within the metaphyseal fragment on the concave side of the deformity in question.

 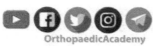

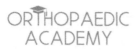

13. During cast application, all of the following are directly related to the risk of thermal injury EXCEPT?

Best answer: **E**
Type of fracture pattern

Explanation:
Overwrapping with fiberglass and placing limb on a pillow decreases the dissipation of heat from the exothermic reaction.

_____

14. Percutaneous ilio-sacral screw placement will have which of the following likely neurologic complication?

Best answer: **C**
Weakness in Great toe extension

Explanation:
Percutaneous Iliosacral screw insertion will probably risk L5 which is responsible to Great toe extension .

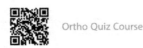
Ortho Quiz Course

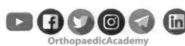
OrthopaedicAcademy

admin@orthopaedicacademy.co.uk
contact@orthopaedicacademy.co.uk

15. The proximal aspect of the posterior approach (Thompson) to the radius involves what surgical interval?

Best answer: **B**

Extensor carpi radialis brevis and extensor digitorum communis

Explanation:

Proximally, the interval is between the ECRB (radial nerve) and the EDC (PIN), whereas more distally, the interval is between the ECRB (radial nerve) and EPL (PIN).

_____

16. Which of the following statements is incorrect regarding ankle fractures?

Best answer: **A**

On a mortise view, the tibiofibular overlap should normally be more than 4mm

Explanation:

On a mortise view, the tibiofibular overlap should normally be more than 1 mm. The mortise ankle view is typically performed with the patient supine and the foot in dorsiflexion. The x-ray beam is directed perpendicular to the ankle joint, and the foot is internally rotated 45 degrees. This rotation helps to bring the talus into profile.

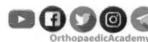

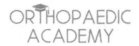

17. When approaching a proximal diaphyseal radius fracture via the Henry approach (volar), the forearm is supinated to minimize injury to what structure?

Best answer: **C**

Posterior interosseus nerve

Explanation:

Forearm should be supinated to move the PIN away from the surgical field.Conversely,in the Thompson(posterior)approach to the forearm, forearm should be pronated to move the PIN away from surgical field

---

18. A child is admitted with a femur shaft fracture. You are considering using Gallows traction to manage this injury. Which of the following is a contraindication for your choice?

Best answer: **C**

There is an ipsilateral humerus fracture

Explanation:

Gallows traction can be used in infants and small children weighing approximately up to 15 kg. Gallows traction can be used in infants and small children weighing approximately up to 15 kg.The child's must hang freely off the bed to ensure the desired line of pull. Vigilant surveillance is imperative due to potential complications including nerve impingement, skin breakdown, and pressure injuries.

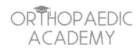
ORTHOPAEDIC ACADEMY

www.orthopaedicacademy.co.uk
www.orthopaedicacademy.net

19. A previously healthy man who weighs 70 kg (154 lb) sustains an acute blood loss of 2 liters after a motorcycle crash. Which of the following statements about physiologic parameters is unique to this amount of blood loss?

Best answer : **D**
Systolic blood pressure will be decreased with a narrowed pulse pressure

Explanation:
A blood loss of 2 liters places the patient in a class IV hemorrhage of more than 40% blood volume loss.

Classification of Hemorrhagic Shock				
	Class I	Class II	Class III	Class IV
Blood Loss (%)	<15%	15-30%	31-40%	>40%
Heart rate	60-100	101-120	121-140	>140
Blood Pressure	Normal	Normal	Decreased	Decreased
Mental status	Slightly anxious	Mildly anxious	Anxious, confused	Confused, lethargic
Fluid requirements	Crystalloid	Crystalloid	Crystalloid, blood products	Crystalloid, blood products

---

20. Which of the following fluoroscopic views is used to assess intra-articular screw penetration during volar fixation of a distal radius fracture?

Best answer: **D**
23° elevated lateral view

Explanation:
Due to radial inclination, a true lateral view of the wrist will not show whether screws from a volar plate are intra-articular; a 23° elevated lateral view is needed to adequately assess this.

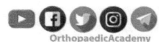

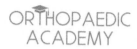
ORTHOPAEDIC ACADEMY

www.orthopaedicacademy.co.uk
www.orthopaedicacademy.net

21. A fracture of the radial head is surgically exposed using a posterolateral approach to the elbow. Once the radial head is exposed, how should the arm be positioned to best protect the posterior interosseous nerve from injury?

Best answer: **D**

Forearm pronation

Explanation:

As long as the dissection stays proximal to the annular ligament, the PIN is not at risk for injury. Forearm pronation ensures that the nerve is as far removed from the surgical field as possible.

---

22. When plating fractures of the femoral diaphysis, the plate should be applied to which surface of the femur?

Best answer: **B**

Posterolateral

Explanation:

Vastus lateralis should be elevated from linea aspera. This exposes the posterolateral surface of femur, which is flat and accommodates a plate well. There is minimal stripping of blood supply.

The plate acts as a tension band when placed laterally, which is the side of the femur that experiences tension during weight bearing. This placement is in accordance with the principle of tension banding in fracture repair, which can help to convert tensile forces into compression forces at the fracture site, promoting healing.

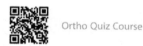
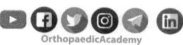

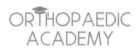

23. Which of the following statements is incorrect regarding ankle fractures?

A - On a mortise view, the tibiofibular overlap should normally be more than 4mm

Explanation:
On a mortise view the tibiofibular overlap should normally be more than 1mm.
The mortise ankle view is typically performed with the patient supine and the foot in dorsiflexion. The x-ray beam is directed perpendicular to the ankle joint, and the foot is internally rotated 45 degrees. This rotation helps to bring the talus into profile.

_____

24. 65-A patient undergoes open reduction and internal fixation of a displaced radial neck fracture. What position should the forearm be in during the approach and during fixation?

Best answer: **C**
Pronated during the approach and neutral for plate application

Explanation:
Pronating the forearm protects posterior interosseous n. Placing the plate straight lateral with forearm in neutral rotation puts the plate in the safe zone that doesnt articulate with proximal RUJ

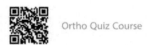
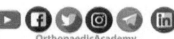

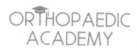

25. What measurement of intracompartmental pressure could help confirm the diagnosis of an acute compartment syndrome in addition to clinical suspicion?

Best answer : **E**
Delta p' of 25 mmHg

Explanation:

Delta p' is defined as the difference between the measured intracompartment pressure and the diastolic blood pressure. A diagnosis of compartment syndrome is supported when the 'delta p' is less than 30 mmHg. Some suggest that an absolute measure of the intracompartmental pressure greater than 30 mmHg also supports the diagnosis. Regardless of finite measurements, high clinical suspicion should always warrant consideration for emergent fasciotomies.

Concise Orthopaedics

To view the book, scan the QR

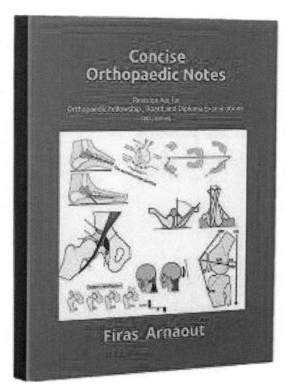

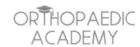
Postgraduate Programme in Musculoskeletal Medicine
To access a course, scan the QR code

Advanced Certificate in the Principles of Orthopedics
To access a course, scan the QR code

Orthopedic X-Ray Interpretation Course
To access a course, scan the QR code

FRCS Case Studies
To access a course, scan the QR code

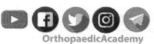

Ortho Quiz Course

OrthopaedicAcademy

admin@orthopaedicacademy.co.uk
contact@orthopaedicacademy.co.uk

Printed in Great Britain
by Amazon